Gluten Free & Fabulous

Over 120 Easy & Delicious
Wheat/Gluten Free Recipes

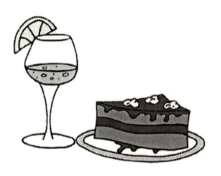

Melanie Martin

This book is dedicated to my husband Tyler, for showing his unconditional love and support in the making of this book by always cleaning up my messy kitchen. ♡

"Among those kinds of food which the good housekeeper should scrupulously banish from her table, is that of hot leavened bread...I believe it more often lays the foundation of diseases of the stomach, than any other kind of nourishment used among us"

-Sarah Josepha Hale
The Good Housekeeper (1839)

Copyright © 2006 by Melanie Martin. All rights reserved.

ISBN 978-1-84728-353-5

Written by Melanie Martin
Cover art by Tyler Martin

Oven Temperatures

Fahrenheit	Centigrade	Gas Mark
225	110	1/4
250	130	1/2
275	140	1
300	150	2
325	170	3
350	180	4
375	190	5
400	200	6
425	220	7
450	230	8
475	240	9

Metric Conversions

1/4 tsp - 1 ml
1/2 tsp - 2 ml
3/4 tsp - 3 ml
1 tsp - 5 ml
1 Tbs - 15 ml
1/4 cup - 60 ml
1/3 cup - 75 ml
1/2 cup - 125 ml
2/3 cup - 150 ml
3/4 cup - 175 ml

1 cup - 250 ml
1 1/4 cup - 300 ml
1 1/2 cup - 375 ml
2 cups - 500 ml
2 1/2 cups - 600 ml
1 oz - 30 grams
3 oz - 85 grams
8 oz - 250 grams
16 oz - 500 grams

Foreword

Seven years ago, after months of chronic pain and malnutrition, I was diagnosed with Celiac disease. I hadn't realized genetic autoimmune conditions that could develop at any age like this, existed. The word "disease" jumped out at me like a ton of bricks smashing me in the face. What a relief to learn it "simply" meant a life-long restricted diet of no wheat, barley, rye or oats (easy, right?). I was just so relieved to learn I wasn't dying of stomach cancer, I would have agreed to eat card-board for the rest of my life at that point! I literally wanted to kiss the doctors feet I was so grateful for the diagnosis.

Celiac disease has many different symptoms, and differs with each individual. Intestinal problems such as bloating, gas, abdominal pain and diarrhea and/or constipation are very common with celiac disease, but there are many other symptoms one may experience as a result of gluten consumption. Some of these include anxiety/panic attacks, hyperactivity, extreme irritability, insomnia, fatigue, infertility and depression, to name a few.

Shortly after being diagnosed I received a couple of gluten free cookbooks as gifts. I remember feeling quite frustrated with these books. I found that the recipes were so long and complicated. I felt very resentful that, in addition to having to drastically change my diet for the rest of my life, I was now, apparently, expected to have the talent and skill to become a gourmet chef over night as well.

I immediately wanted to write a simple cook book for other newly diagnosed celiacs, so they too wouldn't experience the same frustration I felt. However; I didn't know anything about the diet at that point. I, myself, was still eating a can of plain tuna for lunch, as I didn't know what was o.k and what wasn't.

So, several years later, a little older, and a little wiser, I have finally written that book. I don't claim to know it all, but I do know that not every celiac wants to have to be a gourmet chef in order to be able to eat good food.

For the first few years of being celiac, I bought all my gluten free desserts because I was too stubborn, and far too lazy, to bake gluten free. I wanted the same convenience as every body else- to grab, and go.

In recent years however, I started experimenting more in the kitchen and realized, it's really not so hard after all. Homemade products always taste so much better than store bought, and once I realized that, it seemed worth the effort to make my own gluten free cookies and cakes.

That said- I am going to take a break from baking for a little while now, as for the first time in my life, I seem to have somehow acquired a few extra pounds. Now how did that happen?

"It is one of the most beautiful compensations of life, that no man can sincerely try to help another without helping himself"
                              -Ralph Waldo Emerson

Introduction

"Our strength grows out of our weakness"- Ralph Waldo Emerson

The diagnosis of Celiac disease comes as "bitter-sweet" to most new celiacs. "Sweet" is finally having an answer to the reason behind your food related symptoms and suffering, and being able to do something about it. "Bitter" is the fact that life has now changed, becoming slightly more complicated.

The good news is that you are not alone. What used to be referred to as an extremely rare condition is now known to be a very common condition. This means that manufacturers are beginning to take more notice. With every passing year, more and more products are popping up on the market, designed specifically for those on a gluten restricted diet, and this means life keeps getting a little easier for us as time goes on.

Having to switch to a gluten free diet is initially very confusing and overwhelming. Food, for some, becomes downright scary, and some people become afraid to eat, for fear there may be hidden gluten in everything. In the beginning, the best thing a newly diagnosed celiac can do, is to try and stay positive by concentrating on the foods they "can" have, and not the foods they "can't".

Initially, while learning about which products contain gluten and those that don't, it is a good idea to simplify your diet for a little while until your knowledge increases. This may seem a little boring at first, but gradually your diet selection will increase as you learn.

Temporarily, avoid processed, man-made foods, until you are more sure of them, and focus on eating foods in their natural states. Foods such as rice, potatoes, fresh fruit, vegetables and plain meats are a safe bet. For breakfast, foods such as eggs, gluten free toast, or fruit smoothies are a safe choice. There are quite a few gluten free cereals available, as well as pancake and muffin mixes. For lunch, try things like fruit and cheese, salads with a gluten free dressing, gluten free crackers or cookies, and air-popped popcorn.

Introduction

Many people may find they cannot eat the same amounts as they used to without putting on weight more easily, as they are absorbing more nutrients and calories, now that health has been restored. I am reminded of a magnet my mother had on the refrigerator when I was growing up, that said "Eat to live, don't live to eat." This is a good way to view food. It is easier to eat healthier foods when you tell yourself it is by choice and that you want to eat better, for the sake of your health, then to just feel "restricted".

You will be surprised, how over time, your tastes will change and foods that once did not appeal to you, may suddenly become more appetizing, just because you are happy to be able to have them, and add that extra variety to your limited diet.

What once seemed strange to me, now feels very normal. I actually prefer my burgers bun-less now, as that's what I've become accustomed to, although there are gluten free buns available. Another option is to wrap a patty in a large lettuce leaf. Celiac disease is about getting creative, and thinking outside of the box when it comes to food.

There are many gluten free bread products available, although they sometimes tend to be on the dry side, since they are usually stored frozen to maintain freshness. You will most likely find that you prefer to toast these products. It is a good idea to have your own separate toaster as well, to avoid cross contamination from family members' crumbs. Watch out for crumbs in the condiments too- it is a good idea to have your own separate items, as wheat-crumbs in the butter aren't worth getting sick from.

A good sandwich choice, with gluten free bread, is grilled cheese or B.L.T's. Since these are normally toasted anyway, you shouldn't notice much difference. Gluten free bread also makes great french toast- because it is so dry it really absorbs the moisture of the egg mixture. For soft sandwiches I would suggest the gluten free bread mixes, they tend to be softer and fresher.

Baking from scratch, gluten free, is a little more difficult than baking with wheat flour, but with a little practice good results can be achieved. Wheat free flours work best if you combine a few together. This creates a less grainy, better texture. Xanthum gum, or guar gum, found in health food stores need to be used in some baked goods.

These act as a binder, replacing the gluten found in wheat flour, so your product will be moist and not crumbly. Unflavored gelatin is also an option as a binder.

If you ever try to make cookies and they fall apart for some reason, don't throw them out- freeze the crumbs and use later to make a crumb pie crust.

Wheat/gluten is in many things you wouldn't suspect, such as soy sauce. This is why it is important to always read the ingredients on products. You should always read the ingredients every time, even when you buy something you regularly purchase, as sometimes companies change their ingredients.

Most companies have phone numbers on their products and it is easiest, in my opinion, to simply call, and ask if something contains gluten, rather than trying to figure it out for yourself, especially when you are new to the diet.

The most difficult thing about a gluten free diet most celiacs would agree, is eating out at restaurants. If you are lucky enough to live in a big city, you will probably find restaurant staff more knowledgeable about celiac disease, than if you reside in a more rural community, since they may have had more experience with celiac customers.

It is a good idea to always let your server know that you cannot have wheat/gluten even if you are ordering something that you think is o.k. That way, your meal won't show up with a piece of unexpected garlic toast sitting on top of it, or something like that! Remember to ask for your salads with no croutons, and ask for no sauces of any kind to be on anything unless they can guarantee them to be gluten free. If the server is only "pretty sure" something is o.k, I strongly suggest you avoid it.

Be wary of food prepared in common deep fryers, as cross-contamination from crumbs is a possibility. Some fries are bleached with wheat starch, something else to inquire about. I once ate at a restaurant, and got very sick from their nacho's of all things, something I normally can safely eat. It turns out they rolled their grated cheese in flour to prevent it from sticking!

It is a good idea to explain to your server about your dietary restrictions due to being celiac, as you will receive much better service

Introduction

than if they just assume you are being "picky" about your food. Ask them to relay this information to the cook as well.

Try to frequent restaurants at their slower, less popular hours, if possible. They will then be more available to focus on your dietary needs and less likely to rush and screw up your order. The less food being prepared at any given time in a busy commercial kitchen, also reduces your risk of cross-contamination.

Do not put your health in the hands of a stranger, ask many questions to ensure your meal is safe. You do not need to feel embarrassed or afraid to make your needs known to the restaurant staff. You have the right to dine out and not leave ill.

I tend to eat very basically at restaurants now and save my experimentation and variety for when I am preparing food for myself at home. This is just my personal preference, as if I get contaminated I can be affected for up to a month, before feeling completely well again.

Any restaurant with an actual chef is always a good thing, as they usually know a lot about dietary restrictions, and will know everything that has been put in the food, since they usually make it from scratch themselves. They are usually quite good about preparing your food safely, and can also make recommendations from the menu, for you.

There is a lot of information available about Celiac disease, and the gluten free diet. It is a good idea to research it as much as you can, from reliable sources. This will make your life less complicated in the long run. If you have a celiac support group in your city, I highly recommend attending the meetings. It is a great way to meet others like yourself, and educate yourself about staying healthy in a grain filled world. Eventually, it really does get easier! Health and happiness to you.

Contents

Appetizers 7
Beverages 19
Soups 31
Salads 39
Side-dishes 49
Entrees 63
Baked Goods 87
Desserts 93
Miscellaneous 133
Index 142

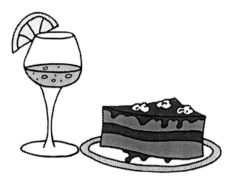

"We are, each of us, angels with one wing and we can only fly by embracing one another"
- Lucian de Creszenza

Gluten Free & Fabulous

Appetizers

Appetizers

Baked Potato Skins

"Let the sky rain potatoes"
- William Shakespeare (1564-1616)
The Merry Wives of Windsor

- scrubbed skins from 2 1/2 lbs Russet potatoes, left in wide strips
- olive oil
- salt
- grated cheddar cheese
- 1 green onion, chopped, optional
- real bacon bits, optional

Scrub potatoes, dry well and prepare skins by scooping out desired amount of potato. Preheat oven to 425°F. Toss skins with some olive oil, coating well. Arrange in a single layer on a baking sheet.

Bake 8 to 12 minutes, or until they are crisp and golden brown. If you are adding cheese, green onions, and bacon bits, top skins with these ingredients half way through bake time. Serve with sour cream for dipping if desired.

-4 servings

Cheddar Cheese Ball

"Tastes are made, not born"
-Mark Twain

- 3 (8 oz) packages cream cheese, softened
- 1 cup sharp cheddar cheese, grated
- 2 tsp onion, minced
- 1 tsp garlic, minced
- 1/4 tsp lemon juice
- 2/3 cup nuts, finely chopped

Flatten cream cheese into mixing bowl. Add the cheddar, onion, garlic and lemon juice and mix together with a large spoon. Form into 2 medium-sized balls, the size of baseballs.

Roll in the finely chopped nuts. Refrigerate overnight, to blend flavors. Serve with gluten free crackers.

Appetizers

Cheese Nachos

"The poets have been mysteriously quiet on the subject of cheese"
    -Gilbert Chesterton

- 1 package gluten free corn tortilla chips
- 1 tomato, chopped
- 2 green onions, chopped
- 1/3 cup black olives, chopped
- 3 cups cheddar cheese, shredded
- chopped chicken, optional

Spread corn chips on an oven safe dish or platter. Sprinkle with tomato, green onions, olives and cheddar cheese. Season to taste. Place under broiler, briefly, until cheese is melted. Serve with sour cream or salsa for dipping.

Note: If desired, add chopped up chicken to this recipe.

-4 servings

Chicken Fingers

> "Eat what you like and let the food fight it out on the inside"
> -Mark Twain

- 3 boneless, skinless, chicken breasts, cut into strips
- 2 Tbs butter or margarine, melted
- 1 cup gluten free corn flake cereal, crushed
- 2 Tbs white sugar
- 1/2 tsp salt
- 1/2 Tbs poultry seasoning
- 2 eggs, lightly beaten
- 3 Tbs honey
- 1 Tbs Dijon mustard

In a shallow bowl, combine the cereal crumbs, sugar, salt and poultry seasoning with the melted butter and set aside. Rinse chicken and pat dry with paper towels. In a separate bowl lightly beat the eggs. Moisten chicken with the beaten eggs, then roll in the crumb mixture, pressing to coat all sides thoroughly. Place on a lightly greased baking sheet and bake at 350°F for around 40 minutes or until tested done.

Note: For the dipping sauce mix together the honey and mustard in a small bowl suitable for dipping. Adjust to preferred taste.

-2 servings

Appetizers

Deli Meat Roll-Ups

"If it looks like a duck and walks like a duck, it probably needs a little more time in the microwave"
-Lori Dowdy

- 1 (8 oz) package of cream cheese, softened
- 1/2 cup chopped olives
- 1/3 cup chopped green onions
- 8 to 10 slices gluten free deli meat of choice (ham is good)

Soften cream cheese by letting sit at room temperature for 15 minutes. Mix together the olives, onions and cream cheese until well blended.

Spread portion of mixture onto meat slice then roll up. Repeat with all slices then refrigerate for 30 to 60 minutes. Cut the rolls into 1/2" rounds. Arrange on a platter with other snacks, such as fresh fruit and cheese cubes.

Deviled Eggs

"Love and eggs are best when they are fresh"
-Russian Proverb

- 6 eggs, hard boiled and peeled
- 1/3 cup gluten free mayonnaise
- 1/4 cup chopped celery
- 1 Tbs gluten free mustard
- paprika to taste
- salt and pepper to taste

Hard boil the eggs and let cool. When cooled, peel and cut in half lengthwise. Carefully remove the yolks with a spoon and set whites aside.

In a medium bowl combine the yolks, mayonnaise, celery and mustard. Add salt and pepper to taste. Spoon egg yolk mixture into egg whites. Sprinkle with paprika. Chill before serving.

-12 servings

Appetizers

Holiday Cheese Truffles

"Strange to see how a good dinner and feasting reconciles everybody"
-Samuel Pepys (1633-1703)

- 16 oz (500 g) cream cheese, softened
- 7 oz (200 g) old or sharp cheddar cheese, shredded
- 1 tsp garlic powder
- dash of ground red pepper
- 1/4 cup roasted red peppers, chopped
- 1/4 cup chopped green onions
- gluten free crackers

Beat cream cheese, shredded cheese, garlic powder and dash of ground red pepper until well blended. Divide in half. Add red peppers to one half and green onions to other half mixing each until well blended. Cover. Refrigerate 2 to 3 hours to allow the flavors to blend.

Shape mixtures into 1-inch balls. Roll in one of these options: finely chopped nuts, grated parmesan cheese, sesame seeds, or chopped fresh parsley. Cover and refrigerate until ready to serve. Serve with gluten free crackers.

-makes 50 truffles

Honey Mustard Chicken Wings

"When having a smackerel of something with a friend, don't eat so much that you get stuck in the doorway trying to get out"
-Winnie the Pooh

- 1 1/2 lbs chicken wings, thawed if frozen
- 1/4 cup liquid honey
- 2 Tbs Dijon mustard

Preheat oven to 375°F. Rinse chicken and pat dry with paper towels. In a large bowl mix together the honey and mustard. Add the chicken wings and mix until well coated.

Arrange wings in a large baking dish and pour remaining mixture overtop. Bake until wings are done, about 30-40 minutes. Serve hot.

Note: For a variation on this recipe substitute the homemade honey sauce with gluten free barbecue sauce.

-4 servings

Appetizers

Parmesan Hummus Dip

"Simplicity is the ultimate sophistication"
-Leonardo Da Vinci

- 1 can (19 oz) chick peas
- 1/2 cup gluten free mayonnaise
- 1/4 cup grated parmesan cheese
- 4 garlic cloves, minced
- 1 Tbs lemon juice
- dash of ground cumin

Place the can of chick peas, drained (reserving 2 Tbs liquid) in a blender or food processor with steel blade. Add in reserved 2 Tbs liquid. Cover and blend until smooth.

Add the mayonnaise, grated parmesan cheese, minced garlic, lemon juice and ground cumin; blend until smooth. Chill. Serve with cut up vegetable slices or gluten free corn chips for dipping.

-makes 2 cups

Smoked Salmon Spread

"Fish and guests in three days are stale"
-John Lyly, author (1554-1606)

- 1 (8 oz) package of cream cheese, softened
- 1/2 cup smoked salmon
- 1/4 cup gluten free mayonnaise
- 3 Tbs finely chopped pecans

Combine cream cheese, smoked salmon, mayonnaise and finely chopped pecans, mixing together well. Chill for several hours, before serving, for the best flavor.

Serve with gluten free crackers. You could also spread this on toasted gluten free bagels.

-4 to 6 servings

Appetizers

Spinach Artichoke Dip

"Men become passionately attached to women who know how to cosset them with delicate tidbits"
-Honorede Balzac (1799-1859)

- 1/2 of a (250g) container of cream cheese
- 1 (10 oz) package of frozen spinach, thawed and drained
- 1 cup shredded mozzarella cheese
- 1/2 cup gluten free mayonnaise
- 2 cloves garlic, minced
- 1/2 cup finely chopped artichoke, optional

Preheat oven to 350°F. Soften cream cheese in microwave, about 30 seconds. In a small casserole dish mix cream cheese, spinach, mozzarella, mayonnaise, minced garlic and artichoke.

Bake in preheated oven for about 20 minutes or until lightly browned. Serve with gluten free corn chips for dipping.

-4 to 6 servings

Beverages

Beverages

Christmas Party Punch

"Christmas is a time when you get homesick, even when you're home"
-Carol Nelson

- 1 cup sugar
- 1 cup water
- 2 (2 ltre) bottles ginger ale
- 4 cups cranberry juice
- 1 cup lemon juice
- 2 cups orange juice
- 2 cups unsweetened pineapple juice

Combine sugar and water in a small saucepan. Bring to a boil stirring until sugar dissolves. Cover and boil over low heat without stirring, for 5 minutes. Add fruit juices and chill. Just before serving put ice in punch bowl and pour in juice mixture. Stir in ginger- ale.

-25 servings

Cranberry Ginger Tea

"There is no trouble so great or grave that cannot be much diminished by a nice cup of tea"
-Bernard Paul Heroux

- 2 tea bags, such as Orange Pekoe
- 2 cups hot water
- 1/2 cup ginger, fresh and thinly sliced
- 1/2 cup cranberries
- 1/2 cup cranberry juice
- pinch of nutmeg

Steep tea, ginger and cranberries in water for 15 minutes. Strain and add nutmeg and cranberry juice. Garnish with cinnamon sticks if desired. Serve warm.

-2 servings

Beverages

Fountain of Youth Smoothie

"Grow old along with me, the best is yet to be"
-Robert Browning

- 1/4 cup skim milk
- 1 cup (8 oz) plain yogurt
- 1 Tbs liquid honey
- 10 fresh strawberries, washed and stems removed
- 1 medium banana
- 1 cup ice cubes

In a blender, puree together the milk, yogurt, honey, strawberries and banana.
Add the ice cubes a couple at a time, blending between additions until smooth. Pour into a tall glass and enjoy.

-1 serving

Iced Cappuccino

"Behind every successful woman...is a substantial amount of coffee"
-Stephanie Piro

- 1 cup gluten free vanilla ice cream
- 1 cup cold strong-brewed coffee
- 2 tsps sugar
- 1 tsp unsweetened cocoa powder
- 1 tsp gluten free vanilla extract

Place all ingredients in blender, blending until smooth. Place container in freezer and freeze for about 1 1/2 hours or until the top and sides of mixture are partially frozen. Scrape sides of container, and process again until smooth and frothy. Serve immediately.

Note: For an "Iced Mocha" increase the unsweetened cocoa to 1 Tbs and proceed as above.

Tip: To add extra flavor to this drink, you could add a dash of ground cinnamon to the coffee grounds before brewing.

-2 servings

Beverages

Mimosa

"Some say the glass is half empty, some say the glass is half full, I say, are you going to drink that?"
-Lisa Claymen

- 3/4 cup champagne, chilled
- 1/4 cup orange juice

Mix together the champagne and orange juice, serve in champagne flutes. This recipe serves two. To adjust amount of servings, mix three parts champagne to one part orange juice.

Note: For kids, make a non-alcoholic version by substituting the champagne with lemon-lime soda.

Tip: For a cranberry mimosa substitute the orange juice with cranberry juice.

-2 servings

Mochaccino

"Coffee leads men to trifle away their time, scald their chops and spend their money, all for a little base, black, thick, nasty bitter, stinking nauseous puddle water"
-The women's petition against coffee (1674)

- 1 cup (8 oz) coffee, brewed double strength
- 2 Tbs sugar
- 2 Tbs unsweetened cocoa powder
- 1 cup milk or dairy substitute
- ground cinnamon to taste

Mix together the sugar and cocoa in a small bowl; divide between two large mugs. Pour 1/2 cup of coffee into each, stirring well to blend.

Next, place milk in a saucepan over medium heat. Using an electric mixer, beat constantly starting at lowest setting and increasing gradually to high, for about 3 minutes or until milk is hot and frothy.

Pour coffee in mugs, spooning foam on top. Sprinkle with ground cinnamon and serve immediately.

-2 servings

Beverages

Orange Smoothie

"Anyone who says sunshine brings happiness has never danced in the rain"
                              -Unknown

- 6 oz can frozen concentrated orange juice
- 1 cup milk or dairy substitute
- 1 cup water
- 1/4 cup white sugar
- 1 tsp gluten free vanilla extract
- 8 ice cubes

Pour the orange juice, milk, water, sugar and vanilla extract into blender. Blend. Add ice cubes one at a time blending between additions. Serve.

Note: You can change the flavor of this smoothie simply by changing the flavor of the juice used. Orange juice makes it taste like the popular Orange Julius.

-3 to 4 servings

Peanut Butter Banana Smoothie

"No man in the world has more courage than the man that can stop after eating one peanut"
-Channing Pollock

- 1 cup milk or dairy substitute
- 2 Tbs gluten free peanut butter (or more if desired)
- 1 ripe banana
- 1/2 tsp ground cinnamon

Place all of the above ingredients in a blender and puree until blended smooth. If desired, a few ice cubes can also be added, one at a time, blending between each addition.

Note: This makes a great quick breakfast or healthy after school snack.

-1 serving

Beverages

Peppermint Hot Chocolate

"Love is like swallowing hot chocolate before it has cooled off. It takes you by surprise but keeps you warm for a long time"
                    -unknown

- 2 squares unsweetened bakers chocolate
- 3 cups milk
- 1 cup water
- 1/4 cup white sugar
- 1 tsp gluten free peppermint extract
- whipped cream or gluten free marshmallows, optional

Heat water and chocolate in saucepan on low heat, stirring constantly with a wire whisk until the chocolate is melted and the mixture is well blended. Add the sugar, then increase the heat to medium high.
Bring to a boil and boil for a few minutes, whisking constantly. Gradually whisk in the milk and peppermint extract. Continue cooking on medium high heat until heated through. Pour into mugs and top with whipped cream or marshmallows if desired.

Tip: At Christmas time add a peppermint candy cane to each mug as a tasty stir- stick.

-3 to 4 servings

Pina Colada

"The problem with the world is everyone is a few drinks behind"
-Humphrey Bogart

- 1 cup ice cubes
- 1 or 2 oz light rum
- 1/4 cup coconut cream
- 1/3 cup pineapple juice
- 1 splash lemon- lime soda
- 1/2 ripe banana

Put the rum, coconut cream, pineapple juice, soda, and banana into a blender and blend well. Slowly add the ice cubes, blending after each addition. Serve in a tall glass. Garnish with a cherry or a fresh pineapple slice if desired.

Note: to make a child friendly version simply omit the rum.

-1 serving

Beverages

Raspberry Iced Tea

"If you are cold, tea will warm you. If you are too heated it will cool you. If you are depressed, it will cheer you. If you are excited it will calm you"
          -William Gladstone

- 2 cups brewed tea, such as Orange Pekoe
- 2 cups raspberry juice
- 1/4 cup liquid honey

Brew two cups of tea and let cool. Mix together the cooled tea, raspberry juice and honey. Whisk until honey is dissolved. Refrigerate. Serve cold with lots of ice.

Note: For a different taste you could substitute the raspberry juice with cranberry juice.

-4 servings

Soups

Soups

Clam Chowder

"In the middle of difficulty lies opportunity"
-Albert Einstein

- 2 Tbs diced bacon
- 3 Tbs butter or margarine
- 2 Tbs chopped onion
- 1 cup boiling water
- 6 cups potatoes, chopped into small cubes
- 1 tsp salt and pepper to taste
- 1 (10 oz) can baby clams with liquid
- 2 1/2 cups milk

In a stove pot, cook the bacon in butter until golden brown and crisp. Add onion and cook until golden. Add boiling water, potatoes, salt and pepper.

Cover. Boil for 15 minutes, stirring occasionally. Add clams with liquid and heat through. Add milk and season to taste. Once soup is heated through, serve immediately.

-6 servings

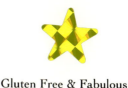

Gluten Free & Fabulous

Hearty Hamburger Soup

"Beef is the soul of cooking"
                -Marie Antoine Careme (1784-1833)

- 1/2 lb ground beef
- 2 Tbs vegetable oil
- 5 tomatoes, peeled and chopped
- 2 cups water
- 6 cups tomato juice
- 1 cup carrots, diced
- 1 cup celery, diced
- 1 1/2 cups onion, diced
- 2 Tbs white sugar
- 1 tsp salt
- 1 tsp each dried basil, thyme and oregano
- 1/2 tsp pepper
- 1 1/2 cups gluten free macaroni noodles

Cook macaroni according to package instructions; drain and set aside. In a large pot, cook ground beef in the oil until meat is thoroughly cooked. Drain meat and return to pot. Combine remaining ingredients, except macaroni. Cover and bring to a boil. Reduce heat and simmer for 30 minutes, or until vegetables are just tender. Add macaroni and cook long enough just to heat through. Serve. Refrigerate leftovers.

Note: If soup is too thick simply add more water. You can add up to two more cups of water without altering the flavor at all.

-10 large servings

Soups

Mom's Chicken Soup

"Too many cooks in the kitchen spoil the soup"
-proverb

- 1 leftover chicken carcass, some meat remaining
- 8 cups of water
- 6 carrots, chopped in 1/2- inch circles
- 8 potatoes, cut into 1/2-inch chunks
- 1 medium onion, diced
- 3 celery spears, chopped in small chunks
- 1/2 tsp salt

Boil chicken carcass in 8 cups of water for 40 minutes. Reduce heat to medium. Remove chicken, set aside to cool. Add carrots, potatoes and onion to pot of broth. Add about 1/2 tsp of salt or to taste. Cook until potatoes and carrots are tender, about 10 minutes. Take remaining chicken off cooled bones and add to soup. Serve hot.

Tip: This soup tastes even better after sitting in fridge overnight.

Note: Add any other seasonings you like to this soup, to suit your tastes.

-4 to 6 servings

Mushroom Soup

"Worries go down better with soup"
-Jewish proverb

- 2 cups mushrooms, chopped
- 2 1/2 cups milk or cream
- 1 gluten free stock cube, dissolved in 2 Tbs hot water
- 2 Tbs butter
- 1 Tbs cornstarch or potato starch
- 1/2 Tbs lemon juice
- 1/4 tsp pepper

Wash mushrooms and cut into slices. Melt butter in a stove pot over medium heat. Add the mushrooms and fry for about 2 minutes. Combine cornstarch with 1/2 cup of milk, stirring until dissolved, and add to the mushrooms.

Gradually stir in the remaining 2 cups milk and stock cube. Add the lemon juice and pepper, then bring to a boil, stirring constantly. Turn heat to low and simmer for about 10 minutes. Serve.

-2 servings

Soups

Potato Leek Soup

"Good manners: the noise you don't make when you're eating soup"
				-Bennett Cherf (1898-1921)

- 3 medium sized leeks
- 1 medium sized onion
- 3 Tbs butter or margarine
- 3-4 medium sized potatoes
- 4 cups gluten free chicken stock
- 1-2 cups milk
- salt and pepper to taste
- chopped chives, optional

Finely chop the onion and white part of the leeks. In a stove pot saute them for a few minutes in the butter. Peel the potatoes and thinly slice. Add the potatoes and chicken stock to the leeks and onion.
Cover and simmer the vegetables for 15 minutes or until tender. Place soup in a blender, blending until smooth. Add milk, salt, pepper and chives. Pour back into soup pot, and heat through. Serve.

-4 servings

Vegetarian Bean Soup

"A man taking basil from a woman will love her always"
-Sir Thomas Moore

- 1 1/2 Tbs olive oil
- 8 green onions, cut into 1-inch pieces
- 2 Tbs garlic, minced
- 5 red bell peppers, cut into thin strips
- 3 cups tomatoes, cut into chunks
- 4 small zucchini, sliced
- 2 squash, thinly sliced
- 1/2 tsp salt
- 1 (19 oz) can kidney beans, rinsed and drained
- 1/2 cup chopped fresh basil or flat leaf parsley
- 1/2 cup water

In a large pot, heat oil over medium high heat. Add green onions and garlic, stirring to mix with oil, and cook for 1 to 2 minutes. Add squash and bell pepper strips, cook 5 to 7 minutes. Add tomatoes and increase heat to high. Cover and cook, stirring often, until tomatoes release juices, about 5 minutes. Stir in zucchini, salt and 1/2 cup water.

Bring to a boil. Reduce heat to medium, cover and cook until vegetables are tender, about 10 minutes. Stir in beans, cover and cook until heated through, 2 to 3 minutes. Sprinkle with chopped basil and serve.

-4 servings

Soups

Yummy Tomato Basil Soup

"Soup of the evening, beautiful..."
                              -Lewis Carroll

- 2 Tbs butter or margarine
- 2 Tbs olive oil
- 4 medium tomatoes, cored and chopped
- 1 small onion, chopped
- 1/4 cup fresh basil, chopped
- salt and pepper to taste
- 2 cups gluten free chicken broth
- 1/2 cup light cream
- 4 sprigs fresh basil for garnish
- shredded mozzarella, optional

Heat the butter and olive oil in a large pot over medium heat. Stir in chopped onion and cook until tender. Mix in chopped tomatoes and chopped basil. Season with salt and pepper. Pour in the chicken broth, reduce heat to low and continue cooking for 15 minutes.

Carefully transfer soup to a blender, or use hand blender, and blend until smooth. Return to the pot and slowly stir in the cream. Cook until heated through. Sprinkle with cheese, if desired, and garnish with fresh basil.

-4 servings

Gluten Free & Fabulous

Salads

Salads

Black Bean Salad

"As a child my family's menu consisted of two choices: take it or leave it"
-Buddy Hackett

- 1 (15 oz) can black beans, rinsed and drained or 1 1/2 cups of freshly cooked black beans
- 1 1/2 cups frozen corn
- 1/2 cup chopped green onions
- 3 fresh plum tomatoes, seeded and chopped
- 1/2 cup fresh chopped cilantro
- 1/4 cup fresh chopped basil
- 2 Tbs lime juice (about juice of 1 lime)
- 1 Tbs olive oil
- 1/2 tsp of white sugar
- salt and pepper to taste

In a large bowl combine the rinsed beans, corn, onion, tomatoes, cilantro, basil, lime juice and olive oil. Add the sugar, and salt and pepper to taste. The sugar helps balance the acidity from the tomatoes and lime. Chill before serving.

-6 to 8 servings

Chef Salad

"Friends are the bacon bits in the salad bowl of life"
-Unknown

- 1 bag mixed salad greens or 6 cups washed lettuce
- 1 or 2 tomatoes, sliced
- 1 cucumber, sliced
- 2 celery sticks, sliced
- 1/2 cup gluten free ham or bacon, cubed or sliced
- 1/2 cup real turkey or chicken, cubed or sliced
- 1 cup cheese, shredded or cubed
- 2 eggs, boiled, peeled and sliced
- real bacon bits, optional

Boil eggs. Set aside to cool. Put everything else in a large salad bowl and gently toss until well mixed.
Peel and slice the cooled eggs and lay slices on top of the salad as a garnish. Drizzle with gluten free salad dressing of choice.

-6 servings

Salads

Cranberry Pecan Salad

"It's so beautifully arranged on the plate, you know someone's fingers have been all over it"
-Julia Child

- 4 boneless, skinless, chicken breasts, cooked and chopped
- 1 bag fancy salad, such as spring mix
- 1 cup pecan pieces
- 1 cup dried cranberries
- 1 cup shredded cheese, such as parmesan
- raspberry vinaigrette dressing

Cook the chicken breasts, cool slightly then chop into cubes. Arrange lettuce on individual plates.

Top with the chicken, pecans, cranberries and cheese. Drizzle with raspberry vinaigrette dressing.

-4 meal size servings

Crunchy Coleslaw

"An onion can make people cry but there's never been a vegetable that can make people laugh"
-Will Rogers

- 4 cups, not packed, of green or purple cabbage
- 1/2 of one carrot, grated very thinly, or chopped
- 2 green onions
- 3 Tbs gluten free mayonnaise
- 1/2 tsp gluten free mustard
- pepper to taste

Thinly slice the cabbage until you have approximately 4 cups of sliced cabbage. Thinly slice a half carrot, as well as the green onions.

Mix the mayonnaise and mustard with the cabbage, carrot and onions. Add pepper to taste. Serve immediately.

-4 servings

Salads

Easy Greek Salad

"To make a good salad is to be a brilliant diplomatist- the problem is entirely the same in both cases. To know exactly how much oil one must put with one's vinegar"
-Oscar Wilde

- 3 medium tomatoes, cut in wedges
- 3/4 of a medium cucumber, halved then cubed
- 1/2 cup feta cheese, crumbled
- 12 Greek olives
- 1/2 cup vinaigrette dressing of choice

In a salad bowl, combine the tomato wedges, cucumber pieces, cheese and olives.
Drizzle with your favorite vinaigrette dressing. Toss well to mix. Refrigerate until ready to serve.

-3 to 4 servings

Fruit and Cheese Summer Salad

"Good thoughts bear good fruit, bad thoughts bear bad fruit"
-James Lane Allen

- 2 cups sliced strawberries
- 2 cups cubed cantaloupe
- 1 cup blueberries
- 1 cup raspberries
- 2 cups cubed havarti cheese
- 1/3 cup orange juice
- 2 Tbs oil
- 2 Tbs liquid honey
- 2 Tbs fresh basil leaves

Combine the fruit and cheese in a large bowl. In a small jar with a tight fitting lid, mix together the orange juice, oil, honey and basil.
Shake vigorously to combine. Pour this mixture over the fruit and cheese and toss well.

-6 servings

Salads

Marinated Veggie Salad

"The embarrassing thing is that the salad dressing is out-grossing my films"
                              -Paul Newman

- 2 tomatoes, cut into wedges
- 1 green pepper, chopped
- 1 orange bell pepper, chopped
- 1 yellow summer squash, thinly sliced
- 1/4 cup minced red onion
- 1/3 cup red wine vinaigrette
- 1 Tbs fresh parsley, minced
- 1 Tbs fresh basil, minced

Combine all vegetables in a salad bowl and stir gently to mix. Combine vinaigrette dressing with parsley and basil and pour over the vegetables.

Mix gently. Let mixture stand at room temperature for one hour to blend flavors.

-6 to 8 servings

Popeyes' Spinach Salad

"It is better to light one candle than to curse the darkness"
-J.R.R. Tolkien

- 4 cups spinach leaves, washed well
- 6 slices bacon, cooked
- 2 hard boiled eggs, sliced
- 2 medium tomatoes, chopped
- 1/2 cup gluten free Ranch salad dressing
- 1 cup cheese, shredded

Wash spinach well, drain and pat dry with paper towels. Tear leaves into bite size pieces, removing stems. Cut tomatoes into wedges. Crumble cooked bacon into pieces.

In a large bowl combine spinach, bacon, tomatoes and sliced eggs. Drizzle with the dressing and sprinkle with cheese.

-4 servings

Salads

Potato Salad

"It is more fun to talk with someone who doesn't use long difficult words, but rather short easy words, like, what about lunch?"
-Winnie The Pooh

- 5 potatoes, boiled
- 5 eggs, hard boiled
- 3 Tbs onion, chopped
- 1 cup gluten free mayonnaise, thinned with milk
- 1/4 cup celery, chopped
- 1/4 cup green pepper, chopped
- 1/4 cup real bacon bits, optional
- salt and pepper to taste

Boil potatoes and let cool. Cut into small squares and place in a large mixing bowl. Boil eggs and let cool. Once cooled, shell, and chop into potatoes. Cut onions into small pieces and add to potatoes. Stir in the celery, green pepper and bacon bits.

Mix one cup mayonnaise with a small amount of milk to thin and stir until smooth. Pour into potatoes and mix well. Add salt and pepper to taste. Chill before serving.

-6 servings

Gluten Free & Fabulous

Side-dishes

Vegetables & Side Dishes

Asparagus With Lemon Butter

"Asparagus inspires gentle thoughts"
-Charles Lamb

- 1 bunch fresh asparagus, washed well
- 2 lemons, for freshly squeezed juice
- 4 oz butter, diced

Squeeze juice from two lemons and heat in a small saucepan over medium low heat. Gradually whisk in the butter, then remove from heat, whisking lightly until thickened.

Serve the sauce at room temperature poured over freshly steamed or boiled asparagus.

-3 to 4 servings

Cheesy Rice Casserole

"In a restaurant, choose a table near a waiter"
-Jewish proverb

- 2 cups rice, uncooked
- 2 tsp salt
- 1 tsp Italian seasoning
- 2 cups grated cheddar cheese
- 1 package frozen spinach, cooked and drained
- 2 Tbs onion, finely chopped
- 1 cup milk
- 4 eggs
- 2 Tbs butter or margarine, melted

Cook rice according to package directions and set aside. Cook spinach according to package directions, drain. Preheat oven to 350°F.

In a large bowl, beat eggs well. Add milk, Italian seasoning and salt to eggs. Fold in the cheese, cooked spinach and cooked rice. Pour into a large, greased casserole dish. Bake for about 35 minutes.

-6 to 8 servings

Vegetables & Side Dishes

Coconut Almond Broccoli

"I do not like broccoli, and I haven't liked it since I was a little kid and my Mother made me eat it, and I'm President of The United States and I'm not going to eat anymore broccoli"
-George Bush

- 2 1/2 cups broccoli florets
- salt and pepper to taste
- 1/2 cup canned coconut cream
- 2 Tbs sliced almonds, toasted

Steam the broccoli uncovered until just tender, about 3 minutes. Drain and sprinkle with salt and pepper. Set aside. In a small pan, warm the coconut cream over medium high heat until it boils, then continue cooking until it reduces by half.

Place broccoli in a serving dish and pour the coconut milk over top. Sprinkle the toasted almonds over top and serve.

-3 to 4 servings

Creamed Corn

"A light wind swept over the corn, and all nature laughed in the sunshine"
-Anne Bronte

- 2 1/2 lbs frozen corn
- 3/4 cup whipping cream
- 1 tsp salt
- 3 tsp white sugar
- 2 tsp cornstarch or potato starch, more if needed

Mix cornstarch with a little bit of the cream and set aside. Meanwhile, place corn in a stove pot over medium heat, along with the salt, sugar and remaining whipping cream.

Bring to a boil. Reduce heat to low or simmer. Thicken with the cornstarch mixture. Heat to desired thickness. Serve.

-4 to 6 servings

Vegetables & Side Dishes

Crunchy Pecan Wild RIce

"Dining is, and always was, a great artistic opportunity"
-Frank Loyd Wright

- 1 cup wild rice, uncooked
- 4 Tbs butter or margarine
- 1 onion, finely chopped
- 1 tsp gluten free seasoning salt
- 1 cup chopped pecans
- 3 Tbs chopped parsley, optional

Prepare wild rice according to package instructions. Saute onion and pecans in butter and sprinkle with the seasoning salt. Stir in the cooked wild rice and cook until heated. Sprinkle with parsley if desired.

Tip: This can be made the day before and reheated in microwave.

-6 to 8 servings

Delicious Rice Stuffing

"A mans' palate can, in time, become accustomed to anything"
-Napoleon Bonaparte (1769-1821)

- 2 cups brown rice, uncooked
- 1/4 cup margarine or butter
- 1 cup onions, chopped
- 1 cup celery, chopped
- 3/4 cup raisons
- 1 1/2 tsp salt
- 3/4 cup walnuts, chopped
- 1/2 tsp poultry seasoning
- 1/2 tsp ground pepper

Cook rice according to package direction and set aside. Cook onions and celery in the margarine until slightly crispy. Blend in the remaining ingredients.

Place in a large, non-greased casserole dish and cover. Bake at 350°F for about 40 minutes, making sure it's heated through.

-8 to 10 servings

Vegetables & Side Dishes

Oven Roasted New Potatoes

"For me a plain roasted potato is the most delicious, it is soothing and enough"
-M.F.K. Fisher (1908-1992)

- 1 1/2 lbs red or yellow new potatoes
- 2 Tbs olive oil
- 2 cloves garlic, minced
- 1-2 tsps fresh rosemary
- 1/4 tsp salt
- pepper to taste

Preheat oven to 450°F. Place potatoes in a mixing bowl. Sprinkle on salt and pepper. Add olive oil, rosemary and garlic. Toss until potatoes are well coated.

Spread potatoes out in a single layer on a baking pan. Roast for about 40 minutes, or until potatoes are cooked through and browned. Serve immediately.

-4 to 6 servings

Stuffed Baked Potatoes

"Heaven is a baked potato and someone to share it with"
-Oprah Winfrey

- 6 potatoes, baked
- 1/2 cup milk
- 1/2 cup fresh parsley, chopped
- 1/2 cup green onions, chopped
- 3/4 cup gluten free sour cream
- 3 Tbs butter
- 2 Tbs cheddar cheese, grated
- 1 tsp paprika
- salt and pepper to taste
- butter, cheese, and paprika; for the topping

Bake potatoes. Let cool enough to handle. Slice potatoes in half lengthwise. Carefully scoop out pulp and beat with other ingredients, with the exception of toppings.

Spread potato mixture back into shells and heat in oven until ready to serve. Top with the butter, cheese and paprika.

-6 to 12 servings

Vegetables & Side Dishes

Sunshine Carrots

"Keep your face to the sunshine and you will not see the shadows"
-Helen Keller

- 1 bag baby carrots
- 1 Tbs brown sugar
- 1 tsp cornstarch or potato starch
- 1/4 tsp ground ginger
- 1/4 cup orange juice
- 2 Tbs butter or margarine

Cook carrots, place in serving dish. In a small saucepan, combine the sugar, cornstarch, ginger and salt. Add orange juice and cook until thickened and boiling.

Remove from heat. Stir in butter. Pour mixture over carrots and serve.

-4 to 6 servings

Sweet Potatoes

"What I say is that, if a man really likes potatoes, he must be a pretty decent sort of fellow"
-A.A. Milne

- 2 medium-size sweet potatoes, scrubbed and dried
- 2 Tbs olive oil
- 2 garlic cloves, minced
- 1 tsp whole cumin seeds
- 1/2 tsp paprika
- salt and pepper to taste

Preheat oven to 500°F. Cut the sweet potatoes in half lengthwise and then in half again. Cut each piece lengthwise into 4 pieces. In a large bowl, toss the sweet potato pieces with the olive oil, garlic, cumin, paprika, salt and pepper, coating well.

Place on a baking sheet and roast them for 20 to 30 minutes or until they are golden brown. Serve immediately.

-4 servings

Vegetables & Side Dishes

The Best Mashed Potatoes

"They (potatoes) are good for boy's cold fingers at suppertime on winter nights"
-Marion Harland
Common Sense in the Household (1873)

- 1 cup shredded cheddar cheese
- 1/3 cup real bacon bits
- 5 medium potatoes, peeled and chopped
- 1 (8 oz) container of gluten free sour cream
- 1 Tbs dried chives, optional

Bring a pot of salted water to a boil. Peel and chop potatoes. Add potatoes to the pot and cook until tender, about 15 minutes. Drain.

Mash potatoes with sour cream. Blend in the cheese and bacon bits. Sprinkle with chives. Season with salt and pepper. Serve while hot.

-8 servings

Zucchini For Two

"Vegetables are a must on any diet. I suggest carrot cake, zucchini bread, and pumpkin pie"
-Garfield

- 2 large tomatoes
- 1 large zucchini
- 1 large green pepper
- 1 medium onion
- 1/2 cup chopped mushrooms, optional
- 1 1/2 Tbs oil

Cut tomatoes into bite sized pieces. Slice zucchini into 1/4- inch round slices. Cut up green peppers into bite size pieces. Slice onion very thinly. Slice up mushrooms. Heat oil in a saucepan and add all vegetables.

Cook on medium heat a few minutes then turn to low and let simmer for around 15 minutes or to desired tenderness. Tomatoes should create a juice.

-2 servings

Vegetables & Side Dishes

Zucchini Parmesan

"The greatest wealth is health"
                                -Virgil

- 4 cups thinly sliced zucchini
- 1 Tbs water
- 1 tsp salt
- 1 small onion, chopped
- 2 Tbs margarine
- fresh ground pepper to taste
- 3 Tbs grated parmesan cheese

Put everything except the cheese in a frying pan. Cover and cook one minute on medium low heat.

Uncover and continue cooking and turning with wide spatula until just tender, about 5 minutes. Sprinkle with the parmesan. Toss well. Serve.

-6 to 8 servings

> Gluten Free & Fabulous

Entrees

Entrees

Adams' Ribs

"To eat is human, to digest divine"
-Mark Twain

- 5 to 7 slabs baby ribs, cut into pieces
- 1 Tbs seasoning salt
- 1 Tbs garlic powder
- 1 tsp cayenne powder, or more to taste
- 1 cup white sugar
- 1/2 cup brown sugar

Boil ribs in water for about 5 minutes. Drain and dry well. In a bowl, mix together the seasoning salt, garlic powder, cayenne powder, and white and brown sugars. Coat ribs with this mixture.

Place coated ribs in roaster, uncovered. Bake at 350°F for about 35 to 45 minutes. Sauce will candy as it cools.

Apple Cinnamon Glazed Chicken

"After a good dinner one can forgive anybody. Even ones' own relatives"
- Oscar Wilde

- 1/3 cup apple jelly
- 1 tablespoon liquid honey
- 1 tablespoon Dijon mustard
- 3/4 teaspoon cinnamon
- 1/4 teaspoon salt
- 4 boneless, skinless chicken breasts

Combine all ingredients, except chicken breasts. Place chicken in casserole dish. Brush mixture onto chicken. Bake for about 30 minutes or until chicken is cooked through. Serve.

Note: Alternately, you could cook on a grill for 15 - 20 minutes, brushing frequently with jelly mixture.

-4 servings

Entrees

Baked Spicy Sweet Ham Slices

"Never eat more than you can lift."
- Miss Piggy, Muppet

- 2 lbs gluten free ham slices, each about 1/2 inch thick
- 1 can (14 oz) crushed pineapple, with juice
- 2 Tbs real maple syrup
- 1/4 tsp ground all spice
- 1/4 tsp ground cloves

Preheat oven to 400°F. Place the ham slices in a baking pan, in a single layer. In a bowl combine the maple syrup, all spice, cloves, and pineapple with juice.

Pour sauce over the ham slices. Bake uncovered for 30 to 40 minutes.

-6 to 8 servings

Barbecue Spiced Tenderloin Steaks

"Life is not merely to live, but to be well"
-Marcus Valerious Martial

- 1 Tbs brown sugar
- 1 Tbs paprika
- 2 Tbs gluten free mustard
- 1 Tbs ground allspice
- 1/4 tsp pepper
- 2 (6 oz) 1-inch thick tenderloin steaks

Combine brown sugar, paprika, mustard, allspice and pepper. Prepare barbecue; high heat. Rub spice mixture generously on both sides of steaks.

Grill to desired state, about 3 minutes per side for medium rare. Serve hot.

-2 servings

Entrees

Brown Sugar Chicken

"There is no love more sincere than the love of food"
-George Bernard Shaw

- 1 1/2 to 3 lbs chicken pieces
- 1 envelope gluten free onion soup mix
- 1/2 cup gluten free ketchup
- 1/4 cup brown sugar
- 1/4 cup water

Preheat oven to 350°F. Place chicken in a single layer on foil in a shallow baking pan. Combine the soup mix, ketchup, sugar and water; pour over the chicken.

Seal edges to make a completely enclosed package. Alternately, you could use a covered casserole dish, but the foil makes for easier clean-up. Bake for about 50 minutes or until chicken is cooked through.

-4 servings

Cheese Stuffed Chicken

"A good meal ought to begin with hunger"
-French proverb

- 4 boneless, skinless chicken breasts
- 1/2 cup crumbled feta cheese
- 3 Tbs fresh parsley, chopped
- 1/2 tsp dried oregano
- 2 Tbs olive oil
- 2 (14 oz) cans tomatoes, undrained
- 1/4 cup sliced black olives
- 1 Tbs corn starch or potato starch

Cut a 3-inch slit in the thick side of each chicken breast to form a pocket, being careful not to cut completely through the flesh. In a bowl, combine cheese, parsley, oregano and oil, mixing gently. Spoon 1/4 of filling into each pocket.

Place chicken in a non-greased baking dish. In another small bowl mix together the tomatoes, olives, and cornstarch and pour over the chicken. Bake at 350°F for 35 to 40 minutes until chicken is thoroughly cooked. Serve.

-4 servings

Entrees

Crock Pot Apple Glazed Pork Roast

"There is one thing more exasperating then a wife who can cook and won't, and that's a wife who can't cook and will"
-Robert Frost

- 4 lb pork loin roast
- salt and pepper to taste
- 6 apples
- 1/4 cup apple juice
- 3 Tbs brown sugar
- 1 Tbs ground ginger

Rub roast with salt and pepper. Brown roast under broiler to remove excess fat; drain well. Core and quarter apples and place in the bottom of the crock pot. Place the roast on top of the apples.

Combine the apple juice, brown sugar and ginger. Spoon over the surface of the roast, covering well. Cover and cook on low, around 6 to 8 hours or until done.

Easy Chili

"Make food simple and let things taste of what they are"
-Maurice Edmond Sailland (1872-1956)

- 1 lb lean ground beef
- 1/3 cup milk
- 1 medium onion, chopped
- 1 Tbs chili powder
- 1 (8 oz) can gluten free tomato sauce
- 1 (16 oz) can kidney beans

Saute beef and onion in a large frying pan. Drain any excess oil. Add the tomato sauce, milk, chili powder and kidney beans. Simmer on low heat for 45 minutes to 1 hour. Serve hot.

-2 to 4 servings

Entrees

Grilled Lemon and Oregano Fish

"Love is a net that catches hearts like a fish"
-Muhammed Ali

- 2 lbs fish steaks, sliced 1-inch thick
- 2 tsp salt
- 4 Tbs lemon juice, preferably fresh
- 2 tsp dried oregano
- 1/2 cup olive oil
- freshly ground pepper to taste

Using a whisk combine the salt and lemon juice in a small bowl until the salt s dissolved. Add the oregano. Whisk in the olive oil in a slow steady stream. Add pepper to taste. Reserve 1/2 of the sauce and marinate fish steaks for 15 to 30 minutes in the remainder.

Grill steaks about 1 to 2 minutes on each side. The surface will not brown. Do not overcook. Place fish on a warm platter and pour the reserved sauce overtop. Serve.

-8 servings

Herbed Salmon Steaks

"I think that fish is nice, but then I think that rain is wet, so who am I to judge?"
-Douglas Adams

- 2 Tbs margarine or butter
- 2 Tbs lemon juice
- 4 salmon steaks, 3/4-inch thick
- 1 tsp onion salt
- 1/4 tsp pepper
- 1/2 tsp dried thyme or marjoram leaves
- paprika to taste
- lemon wedges
- parsley

Place margarine and lemon juice in a 12 x 7-inch baking dish and heat at 400°F. Coat both sides of fish with lemon butter and place in baking dish.

Sprinkle with seasonings and bake uncovered, about 25 minutes or until fish flakes easily with a fork. Sprinkle with paprika, and serve with lemon wedges and parsley.

-4 servings

Entrees

Honey Garlic Chicken

"What garlic is to food, insanity is to art"
                        -Augustus Saint-Gaudens

- 2 Tbs oil
- 2 Tbs liquid honey
- 1 Tbs lemon juice
- 1/3 cup gluten free soy sauce
- 1 tsp fresh ginger root or 1/2 tsp ground
- 1 clove garlic, minced
- 1 Tbs chopped green onion
- 1 1/2 lbs chicken pieces

    Combine all ingredients except the chicken. Marinate the chicken in this mixture for several hours. Remove chicken from marinade.
    Place chicken in baking dish and bake at 350°F for about 45 minutes, using marinade to baste chicken during the last 30 minutes.

    -3 to 4 servings

Lemon Parsley Halibut

"Give a man a fish and he has food for a day; teach him how to fish and you can get rid of him for an entire weekend"
  -Zenna Schaffer

- 1 Tbs unsalted butter
- 1 1/2 1bs halibut steaks,thawed if frozen
- 2 Tbs lemon juice
- salt and pepper to taste
- 2 Tbs parsley, finely chopped
- 1 lemon, cut into wedges

Melt butter in a heavy non-stick skillet over medium heat. Arrange halibut steaks in skillet. Drizzle with lemon juice and season with salt and pepper.

Cover the skillet and simmer for about 8 to 10 minutes or until the fish flakes easily. Sprinkle with parsley and serve with lemon wedges on the side.

-4 servings

Entrees

Manhattan Meatballs

"I didn't fight my way to the top of the food chain to be a vegetarian"

- anonymous

- 1 lb lean ground beef
- 1 cup fresh gluten free bread crumbs
- 1/4 cup onion, chopped
- 1 egg, beaten
- 1 tablespoon parsley, chopped
- 1 teaspoon salt
- 1 tablespoon margarine
- 3/4 cup apricot jam
- 1/4 cup gluten free barbecue sauce

Mix meat, crumbs, onion, egg, parsley and salt in a good sized bowl. Shape into 1- inch meatballs. Heat margarine in a skillet, add meatballs, cooking until browned. Drain and place in casserole dish.

Mix together the jam and barbecue sauce and pour over the meatballs. Bake at 350°F for 30 minutes or until heated through, stirring occasionally. Serve over rice.

-Makes 2 1/2 dozen meatballs

Maple Syrup Chicken

"People who count their chickens before they are hatched, act very wisely, because chickens run about so absurdly that it is impossible to count them"
-Oscar Wilde

- 1 whole chicken, about 3 1/2 lbs, cut into pieces
- 1/2 tsp lemon rind
- 2 tsp fresh lemon juice
- 1/2 cup margarine, melted
- 1/2 cup pure maple syrup
- salt to taste
- 1/4 cup onion, chopped

Place the chicken pieces in a baking pan. In a bowl, mix together the lemon rind and lemon juice, melted margarine, maple syrup, salt and chopped onion.

Pour this mixture over the chicken. Bake at 400°F for 50 to 60 minutes, basting frequently, until done.

-4 servings

Entrees

Orange Zest Salmon

"Why does Sea World have a restaurant? I'm halfway through my fish burger and I realize, oh my gosh...I could be eating a slow learner"
-Lynda Montgomery

- 1 salmon fillet, about 1 1/2 lbs
- olive oil
- salt and pepper to taste
- 1/2 cup gluten free mayonnaise
- 1 Tbs minced orange zest
- 2 Tbs chopped fresh cilantro
- 2 garlic cloves, minced
- 1/2 tsp ground cumin

Rub salmon with the olive oil and place on a lightly oiled sheet pan. Sprinkle with salt and pepper. Set aside. In a small bowl combine the mayonnaise, orange zest, cilantro, garlic and cumin. Adjust the oven rack to sit 3-inches away from broiler heat, and preheat broiler.

Spread the mayonnaise mixture over the salmon in a thin layer. Broil about 7 minutes, or until the fish is cooked through. Serve warm.

-4 servings

Oven-Crisped Pork Chops

"There is poetry in a pork chop to a hungry man"
-Philip Gibbs

- 4 cups gluten free corn flake cereal, crushed
- 1 egg
- 1 Tbs water
- 1 tsp dried oregano
- 1/2 tsp salt
- 1/4 tsp pepper
- 1/4 tsp garlic powder
- 6 thick, centre cut, loin pork chops

In a shallow dish or pan, place crushed cereal and set aside. In a small bowl, lightly beat together the egg, water, oregano, salt, pepper and garlic powder.

Dip the chops into egg mixture. Coat with the crushed cereal and place in a single layer in a lightly greased shallow baking pan.

Bake at 350°F for about 45 minutes or until tender. Do not cover pan or turn pork chops while baking.

-6 servings

Entrees

Parmesan Chicken

"Food is an important part of a balanced diet"
-Fran Leibowitz

- 2 lbs bone-in chicken breasts or thighs
- 1/2 cup gluten free Italian dressing
- 1/2 Tbs Italian seasoning
- 1/2 cup parmesan cheese, grated
- salt and pepper to taste

Heat oven to 400°F. Place chicken pieces in a 9x13-inch baking pan. Pour Italian dressing over the chicken.
Sprinkle evenly with the Italian seasoning and grated cheese. Bake for about 45 minutes until chicken is cooked through.

-4 servings

Pineapple Chicken

"Hunger is the best sauce in the world"
-Cervantes

- 2 to 3 lbs chicken, cut into serving pieces
- 1 Tbs gluten free soy sauce
- 1/2 tsp brown sugar
- 1 Tbs corn starch or potato starch
- 1/4 tsp ground ginger
- 1 (8 oz) can pineapple chunks, including liquid

Heat oil in skillet and brown chicken. Combine sauce ingredients in a separate sauce pan and cook over medium heat, stirring occasionally until thickened.

Pour the sauce over the chicken and simmer until the chicken is cooked through and tender. Serve over rice.

-4 servings

Entrees

Simple Sweet and Sour Chops

"Don't take advice from a butcher on how to cook meat. If he knew he'd be a chef"
-Andy Rooney

- 1/2 cup brown sugar
- 1/2 cup gluten free ketchup
- 1/2 cup water
- lemon slices, one per chop
- 4 to 8 pork chops

Preheat oven to 350°F. Slice lemon and put a lemon slice on each pork chop, set aside. In a bowl, mix together the sugar, water and ketchup.

Pour this sauce over the pork chops. Bake for around one hour, depending on the thickness and number of pork chops.

-4 to 8 servings

Spiced Chicken

"Small cheer and great welcome makes a merry feast"
- William Shakespeare (1564-1616)

- 1 Tbs paprika
- 1 1/2 tsp ground cumin
- 1/8 tsp cayenne pepper
- 8 chicken thighs
- salt and pepper to taste
- 1/4 cup olive oil
- 3 Tbs lemon juice

In a small bowl mix together the paprika, cumin and cayenne pepper. Place chicken piece in a baking dish and sprinkle with salt and pepper. Rub the spice mixture into the chicken.

In a separate bowl, whisk together the olive oil, garlic and lemon juice. Pour over the chicken, turning to cover completely. Place in refrigerator to marinate for several hours or overnight.

Bring to room temperature before baking. Preheat the oven to 400°F. Bake, skin down, for about 20 minutes, turn over, and bake for another 20 minutes or until cooked through and crisp.

-4 servings

Entrees

Sweet and Spicy Chicken

"A great way to lose weight is to eat naked in front of a mirror. Restaurants will almost always throw you out before you can eat too much"
-Frank Varano

- 6 to 8 chicken legs
- 1/2 cup orange marmalade
- 2 tsp chili powder

Preheat oven to 400°F. Line a baking sheet with foil. Combine marmalade and chili powder in a zip-lock bag. Place chicken in bag and gently coat.

Place the coated chicken on baking sheet and spoon any remaining mixture over the chicken. Bake for 30 minutes or until the chicken is fully cooked and tender.

-4 servings

Tarragon Chicken

"I cook with wine. Sometimes I even add it to the food"
-W.C. Fields

- 2 Tbs unsalted butter
- 1 Tbs vegetable oil
- 4 boneless, skinless, chicken breasts
- 3/4 cup dry white wine or apple juice
- 2 tsp Dijon mustard
- 1 Tbs fresh tarragon, chopped, or 1 tsp dried
- salt and pepper to taste
- 3/4 cup heavy cream

Melt butter in a heavy non-stick skillet over medium- high heat. Saute chicken breasts until lightly browned, about 4 minutes per side. Remove chicken, set aside. Add wine to the same skillet. Bring to a boil, scraping up brown bits from bottom of pan with a wooden spoon.

Stir in mustard, tarragon, salt and pepper. Whisk in cream and boil for about 3 minutes or until mixture thickens slightly. Return chicken to pan and turn to coat with sauce. Simmer 5 to 10 minutes, until chicken is tender and cooked though. Serve chicken with sauce.

-4 servings

Entrees

Yummy Lasagna Casserole

"When the lasagna content in my blood gets low, I get mean"
-Garfield

- 2 cups uncooked gluten free Rotini pasta, or pasta of choice
- 1/2 lb lean ground beef
- 1 cup (250 g) cottage cheese
- 1 (14 oz) can gluten free pasta sauce
- 1/2 cup shredded fresh basil leaves
- 1 1/2 cups mozzarella cheese, shredded

Cook pasta noodles according to package directions; drain, set aside. In a frying pan, cook ground beef until fully browned; drain. In a large bowl stir together the cooked pasta, ground beef, cottage cheese, pasta sauce, basil leaves and 1 cup of the shredded cheese.

Place mixture in an 8x8-inch casserole dish, and sprinkle remaining 1/2 cup of cheese overtop. Bake at 350°F, about 15 minutes or until heated through.

Note: if desired you could also add cooked spinach or chopped up, cooked zucchini .

-4 servings

Gluten Free & Fabulous

Baked Goods

Baked Goods

Brazilian Cheese Buns

"Bread, milk, and butter are of venerable antiquity. They taste of the morning of the world"

-Leigh Hunt (1784-1859)

- 1/3 cup olive oil
- 1/3 cup water
- 1/3 cup milk
- 1 tsp salt
- 2 cups tapioca starch
- 2 eggs
- 2/3 cup cheese, shredded (parmesan or cheddar)
- 1/2 tsp garlic powder, optional

Preheat oven to 350°F. In a large metal bowl, or a bowl that can handle heat, place the two cups of tapioca starch and set aside. In a saucepan heat the oil, water, milk and salt bringing it to a boil. As it comes to a full boil it will get white and foamy. At this point pour the mixture into the tapioca starch and mix really well with a wooden spoon. Let cool for about 15 minutes.

Add eggs and cheese, mixing well. It will be sticky. Drop by heaping tablespoons onto a non-greased cookie sheet. Bake for about 25 minutes or until tops are slightly browned.

Note: These are best served warm from the oven, they harden overnight. In Brazil these are called Quejo's and are eaten for breakfast with jam or cream cheese, or as snacks. They have a very chewy texture, which may take some getting used to.

Tip: 1/4 cup mashed potatoes added to dough mixture makes these fluffier, if you prefer.

-12 small rolls

Corn Muffins

> "Kissing don't last, cookery do"
> -George Meredith

- 4 eggs, separated
- 1/2 cup milk
- 1/2 tsp salt
- 1 cup Cream Of Rice hot cereal, uncooked
- 1 (8 oz) can whole kernel corn, drained
- 2 Tbs butter, melted
- 1 Tbs gluten free baking powder
- 2 Tbs white sugar

Separate eggs, setting aside the whites. Beat egg yolks, milk and salt in a medium bowl with a wire whisk until blended well. Add the dry rice cereal and mix well. Let stand for 10 minutes. Preheat oven to 350°F.

Stir corn, melted butter and baking powder into first mixture, set aside. Beat egg whites in a separate medium bowl with electric mixer on high speed until foamy. Gradually add sugar, beating until stiff peaks form. Add to cereal mixture and stir gently until blended well.

Spoon 2 Tbs each into 12 greased or paper-lined medium muffin cups. Bake 18 to 20 minutes or until inserted toothpick comes out clean.

-12 muffins

Baked Goods

Cheesy Pizza Crust

"You better cut the pizza in four pieces because I'm not hungry enough for six"
                            -Yogi Berra

- 2/3 cup brown rice flour
- 1/2 cup tapioca flour or tapioca starch
- 1 Tbs gluten free dry yeast
- 2 tsp xanthum gum
- 1 tsp unflavored gelatin
- 1/2 tsp salt
- 2/3 cup warm milk
- 1/2 tsp liquid honey
- 1 tsp olive oil
- 1 tsp Italian seasoning
- 1/2 cup cheddar cheese, shredded

Preheat oven to 425°F. In a large bowl, blend together the yeast, flours, salt, xanthum gum, gelatin and seasoning. Then add milk, oil, honey and cheese. Knead by hand for a few minutes until a nice consistency is reached.

Grease a 12-inch pizza pan really well. Spread dough out on pan, pressing to cover, keeping it slightly thicker around the edges. Bake crust for 15 minutes. Remove. Top with favorite gluten free sauce and toppings. Bake for about 15 minutes longer.

Note: if pizza sticks to pan, let cool a little bit before trying to remove.

-makes one 12-inch pizza crust

Gluten Free & Fabulous

Potato Flat Bread

"In order to change we must be sick and tired of being sick and tired"

-unknown

- 3 oz (1/3 cup) mashed potatoes, cooked
- 1 egg
- 1/2 cup milk
- 1 oz (2 1/2 Tbs) olive oil
- 1/2 tsp salt
- 1 tsp sugar, optional
- 6 oz (3/4 cup) brown rice flour
- Italian seasoning to taste

Preheat oven to 430°F. In a large bowl beat together the mashed potatoes, egg, milk, oil, salt and sugar. Add the brown rice flour . Mix well but do not over beat. Line the bottom of a rectangular 2 lb loaf tin with parchment paper. Pour in mixture. Sprinkle with Italian seasoning. Bake for 35 to 40 minutes. When tested it should be moist but not raw. Invert onto wire rack to cool.

Note: This bread is best eaten the same day, as it does not keep well. It is a good bread for dipping in oil and balsamic vinegar, or buttered. To safe time, use instant mashed potatoes.

-makes 1 flat bread

Baked Goods

Simply Nutty Banana Bread

"When baking, follow directions, when cooking go by your own taste"
-Laiko Bahrs

- 1 cup very ripe mashed bananas
- 3/4 cup white sugar
- 1 tsp gluten free vanilla extract
- 2 eggs
- 1 1/4 cup white rice flour
- 1/4 cup chopped nuts
- 3/4 tsp gluten free baking powder
- 1/2 tsp baking soda
- 1/4 tsp salt
- 1/4 cup olive oil

Combine the bananas, sugar, and vanilla in a medium bowl and beat on medium speed for 1 minute. Add the eggs and mix well. Combine the rice flour, nuts, baking powder, baking soda and salt in a large bowl. Add the banana mixture and oil to the dry ingredients, mixing well at low speed.

Preheat oven to 350°F. Pour the batter into an 8x4-inch loaf pan. Bake for 50 to 60 minutes or until done. Cool for 5 minutes before removing from pan. Freeze leftovers.

Note: Alternately, you could make banana bread muffins, adjusting cooking time accordingly.

-1 loaf

Desserts

Desserts

Almond Pecan Cake

"Birthdays are nature's way of telling us to eat more cake"
-unknown

- 4 eggs
- 3/4 cup white sugar
- 1/2 cup finely ground almonds
- 1/2 cup finely ground pecans
- 2 Tbs cornstarch or potato starch
- 1 1/2 tsp gluten free baking powder

Preheat oven to 350°F. Grease two 8- inch layer pans. Line with parchment paper. In a bowl, beat eggs and sugar until light and frothy. Add finely ground nuts, cornstarch and baking powder, beating in well. Pour into the prepared pans, the batter will be thin.

Bake for 15 to 20 minutes. Cool for 10 minutes. Line a cookie sheet with wax paper. Turn cakes out onto cookie sheet. Place in freezer for about 20 minutes, this will make it easier to frost. Frost the bottom layer with gluten free icing, cover with top layer and frost as well.

Note: This cake is also good layered with whipped cream and sliced strawberries. Refrigerate this cake.

Apple Crumble

"It was not the apple on the tree but the pair on the ground that caused the trouble in the garden"
                                                              -unknown

- 5 to 6 apples, cored and cut into wedges
- 1/2 cup gluten free flour
- 1/2 cup brown sugar, packed
- 1/2 cup butter
- 1/2 cup nuts, coarsely chopped
- 1/2 tsp cinnamon or more to taste
- 1/2 tsp nutmeg, optional

Preheat oven to 350°F. Place the prepared fruit in an 8x8-inch baking pan. In a medium bowl mix the gluten free flour, sugar, butter and cinnamon. Add nuts, tossing to mix.

Spread this mixture evenly over the fruit. Bake for about 45 minutes or until fruit is cooked. You can serve this warm or cold, plain, or with whipped cream or gluten free ice cream.

Note: You can substitute other fruit for the apples, but if you use canned, make sure to drain really well before using. Fresh "blackberry" crumble is always good.

Desserts

Babe Ruth Bars

"Never let the fear of striking out get in your way"
-George Herman "Babe Ruth"

- 1 cup chunky gluten free peanut butter
- 1 cup white corn syrup
- 1/2 cup packed brown sugar
- 1/2 cup white sugar
- 6 cups gluten free corn flakes cereal
- 1 cup gluten free semi-sweet chocolate chips

In a large saucepan over medium heat, combine the peanut butter, corn syrup, brown sugar and white sugar. Cook, stirring occasionally until smooth.

Remove from heat and quickly mix in the corn flake cereal and chocolate chips until evenly coated.

Press the entire mixture gently into a buttered 9x13-inch baking dish. Allow to cool completely before cutting into bars.

Note: If desired, while still warm, melt more chocolate over top. This gives them a nicer appearance.

Baked Cinnamon Apples

"All millionaires love a baked apple"
-Ronald Firbank (1886-1926)

- 4 tart apples, cored and cut into small chunks
- 2 Tbs butter, diced in small pieces
- 1 Tbs dark brown sugar
- cinnamon to taste

Preheat the oven to 400°F. Place the apple chunks in an 8-inch glass baking dish. Dot with the butter and sprinkle with the brown sugar and cinnamon.

Bake for 30 minutes or until done, stirring once after the first 15 minutes. Serve warm or at room temperature, with whipped cream or gluten free vanilla ice cream if desired.

-4 servings

Desserts

Basic Cheesecake

"Cooking is like love, It should be entered into with abandon or not at all"
-Harriet Van Horne

- 1 1/2 cups gluten free cookie crumbs
- 1 (14 oz) can sweetened condensed milk (not evaporated milk)
- 1/4 cup butter or margarine, melted
- 3 eggs
- 2 tsp gluten free vanilla extract
- 3 (8 oz) packages of cream cheese, softened

Preheat oven to 300°F. Combine gluten free cookie crumbs and butter or margarine. Press into a 9x13-inch baking pan and set aside. In a large mixing bowl, beat the cream cheese until fluffy. Gradually add in the condensed milk. Add eggs and vanilla; blend.
Pour into prepared baking pan. Bake for 20 minutes or until cake springs back when touched. Let cool. Keep refrigerated.

Tip: Serve plain, or top with gluten free pie fillings.

Note: My favorite topping is "almond praline": combine 1/3 cup dark brown sugar and 1/3 cup whipping cream and heat in a saucepan, until sugar melts, then simmer until thickened, about 5 minutes. Remove from heat; stir in chopped, toasted almonds. Spoon evenly over cake.

Berry Lemon Mousse Parfait

"We all live with the objective of being happy; our lives are all different and yet the same"
-Anne Frank

- 3/4 cup whipping cream
- 1/4 cup white sugar
- 1 Tbs lemon juice
- 1/2 tsp gluten free vanilla extract
- 1/2 cup sliced strawberries
- 1/2 cup fresh blueberries

In a large, chilled mixing bowl, using an electric mixer, beat cream, sugar, lemon juice and vanilla until mixture mounds softly. Spoon a layer of fruit into 4 individual dessert dishes, then a layer of whipped topping, and repeat.

Serve immediately or keep chilled for several hours before serving. You could substitute the strawberries and blueberries with raspberries and blackberries if desired.

-4 servings

Desserts

Caramel Bananas

"Nature magically suits a man to his fortunes, by making them the fruit of his character"
-Ralph Waldo Emerson

- 1 cup brown sugar
- 3 Tbs butter or margarine
- 2 Tbs cream
- 1/8 tsp gluten free vanilla extract
- 3 medium bananas, sliced
- 1/2 cup whipping cream
- 1 tsp white sugar
- 1/2 tsp gluten free vanilla extract

In a saucepan, combine the brown sugar, butter, cream and the 1/8 tsp vanilla extract. Bring to a boil over medium heat. Turn heat to low and simmer slowly to let mixture thicken a little bit.

Slice bananas into four individual dessert dishes. Whip the cream, sugar and 1/2 tsp vanilla until soft peaks form. Spoon hot topping over bananas and top with whipped cream.

-4 servings

Chocolate Almond Cupcakes

"A messy kitchen is a happy kitchen and this kitchen is delirious"
-unknown

- 5 large eggs, separated
- 1/2 tsp lemon juice or 1/8 tsp cream of tartar
- 6 Tbs butter or margarine
- 1 tsp gluten free vanilla extract
- 3/4 cup white sugar
- 2 cups finely ground almonds or ground nuts of choice
- 5 Tbs unsweetened cocoa powder
- 2 tsp gluten free baking powder

Line a 12 cup muffin pan with cupcake papers. Preheat oven to 325°F. Beat together the egg whites and lemon juice until they form soft peaks. In another bowl, cream together the yolks, butter, vanilla and sugar until fluffy. Add half the egg whites to the mixture, as well as one cup of the nuts and all of the cocoa and baking powder, stirring in well.

Blend in the remaining egg whites and nuts. Fill the cupcake cups 3/4 full and bake for around 20 minutes, or until slightly cracked on top. Let pan cool on wire rack. Frost and decorate as desired, with your favorite gluten free icing and/or gluten free sprinkles.

-12 cupcakes

Desserts

Chocolate Cake Cookies

"And above all...think chocolate"
    -Betty Crocker

- 1 gluten free chocolate cake mix
- 1/3 cup gluten free sour cream
- 3 Tbs milk
- 1/4 tsp gluten free vanilla extract
- one egg

Preheat oven to 350°F. Lightly grease cookie sheets. In a large bowl combine dry cake mix, sour cream, milk, vanilla and egg. Stir until well blended.

Drop by the tablespoon two inches apart on cookie sheets. Bake for 10 minutes. Let cool for 1 minute before carefully removing from cookie sheets with spatula.

Tip: These should be stored frozen to maintain freshness.

- about 24 cookies

Chocolate Cake Pudding

"All I really need is love, but a little chocolate now and then doesn't hurt"
-Lucy, by Charles M. Schulz

- 1 cup gluten free chocolate chips
- 2 Tbs white sugar
- pinch of salt
- one egg
- 2 Tbs gluten free liquor, optional
- 2/3 cup boiling milk

Place chocolate chips, sugar, salt and liquor in blender. Next, bring milk to a boil over medium heat on stove top. Pour boiled milk into blender over top of other ingredients. Puree until smooth and mixed.

Pour into four individual dessert dishes. Refrigerate for 30 minutes. Serve with whipped cream on each, if desired.

Note: This is a rich, decadent dessert.

Tip: You can freeze this pudding for a cool treat.

-4 servings

Desserts

Chocolate Chip Cookies

"Friends are the chocolate chips in the cookies of life"
-Robin Brewer

- 1/4 cup margarine, softened, not melted
- 3/4 cup brown sugar
- 1/3 cup white sugar
- 2 tsp gluten free vanilla extract
- one extra large egg
- 1 cup flour blend- recipe below
- 1/2 tsp baking soda
- 2 tsp xanthum gum or 4 tsp unflavored gelatin
- 1/4 tsp salt
- 1 1/2 cups gluten free chocolate chips

RICE FLOUR BLEND:
- 3 cups brown rice flour
- 1 1/4 cups potato starch or corn starch
- 3/4 cup tapioca flour or tapioca starch

Preheat oven to 350°F. Use electric mixer to beat margarine, sugars and vanilla until smooth. Beat in egg. In a separate bowl, whisk together one cup of the flour mix, baking soda, xanthum gum and salt. Beat into egg mixture on low speed. Stir in chocolate chips. Drop by tablespoons onto non-stick cookie sheet lined with parchment paper. Bake for 10 to 12 minutes or until cookies are slightly browned. Cool on rack.

Note: Store cookies in airtight container or freeze. Store remaining rice flour blend in airtight container in fridge for future use.

-about 24 cookies

Chocolate Dipped Ice Cream

"Ice cream is exquisite. What a pity it isn't illegal"
-Voltaire (1694-1778)

- 14 oz (450 g) good quality gluten free ice cream
- 11 oz (350 g) semi-sweet chocolate

Line a baking tray with parchment paper. Soften the ice cream slightly by leaving in the fridge for about 10 minutes. Once softened, use a small ice cream scoop to shape the ice cream into small balls. Place the balls on prepared tray and place in freezer until frozen.

Break the chocolate into small pieces and place in a heat proof bowl. Set the bowl over a saucepan of almost boiling water. Stir occasionally until smooth and melted. Cool slightly, but do not let set.

Using two spoons, dip each ice cream ball into the chocolate one by one. Return the chocolate balls to the freezer until ready to serve.

-6 servings

Desserts

Chocolate Dipped Pecan Bites

"Forget love...I'd rather fall in chocolate"
-unknown

- 1 cup finely ground pecans
- 1/3 cup white sugar
- 1 tsp gluten free vanilla extract
- 1 egg white, lightly beaten
- 2 squares semi-sweet baking chocolate, melted

    Lightly beat egg white and set aside. Combine ground pecans and sugar in a bowl. Stir in vanilla. Slowly stir in egg white, stirring until a thin dough forms. Cover and chill for at least 2 hours.
    Heat oven to 350°F. Lightly grease a baking sheet. Measure 16 heaping teaspoonfuls of nut dough and roll each into a ball. Bake 8 to 10 minutes. Cool completely then dip tops in melted chocolate. Store refrigerated.

-makes 16

Chocolate Marshmallow Truffles

"There's nothing better than a good friend, except a good friend with chocolate"
-Linda Grayson

- 1 (250g) package of gluten free marshmallows
- 1 (700g) package gluten free chocolate chips, melted
- 2/3 cup chopped almonds

Melt chocolate then dip marshmallows one at a time, turning to evenly coat each one. Gently shake off any excess chocolate.

Place marshmallows in a single layer, on sheets of wax paper. Sprinkle each with about one teaspoon of chopped almonds.

Place in fridge for 1 to 2 hours or until chocolate hardens. Store in airtight container at room temperature.

-20 servings

Desserts

Chocolate Mousse Pie

"Seize the moment. Remember all those women on the Titanic who waved off the dessert cart"
                    -Erma Bombeck

- 2 cups chopped pecans
- 1/4 cup butter, melted
- 1/4 cup brown sugar
- 1 (8 oz) package of cream cheese, softened
- 1/3 cup unsweetened cocoa
- 1 cup superfine white sugar
- 1/2 cup gluten free vanilla extract
- 2 cups whipping cream
- 2 Tbs superfine white sugar

Preheat oven to 375°F. In a medium bowl, combine nuts, brown sugar and butter, mix well. Press into a 9-inch pie pan. Bake for 8 minutes or until just set. Cool on wire rack. In a large bowl, combine softened cream cheese, cocoa, and one cup superfine sugar. Beat until smooth and fluffy. Add melted chocolate chips and vanilla; beat until smooth.

In a medium bowl, combine whipping cream and the 2 Tbs superfine sugar until stiff peaks form. Beat remaining whipped cream into chocolate mixture to combine. Pour into cooled pie shell. Cover and chill until firm, about 4 to 6 hours.

-8 servings

Chocolate Peanut Cups

"Nothing takes the taste out of peanut butter quite like unrequited love"
-Charlie Brown

- 2 Tbs corn syrup
- 1/4 cup brown sugar
- 1/4 cup gluten free peanut butter, smooth or crunchy
- 2 Tbs butter, melted
- 2 cups gluten free crispy rice cereal
- 1/4 cup peanuts, finely chopped
- 3 oz gluten free semi-sweet chocolate
- 1/2 cup gluten free peanut butter, smooth or crunchy
- 36 peanut halves

Combine corn syrup, 1/4 cup peanut butter, brown sugar and melted butter. Stir in crispy rice cereal and 1/4 cup finely chopped peanuts. Press into the bottoms of 12 well-greased muffin cups. Bake at 375°F for 5 to 8 minutes. Let cool 5 minutes and remove from pan.

Melt chocolate over low heat. Blend in remaining 1/2 cup peanut butter and stir over low heat, until smooth. Spread on top of each cereal cup, spreading almost to edges. Garnish each peanut cup with 3 peanut halves. Refrigerate covered, until serving.

Note: make sure peanuts are gluten free, I have heard sometimes peanuts are bleached with wheat starch.

-12 servings

Desserts

Chocolate Puffed Rice Squares

"Chocolate is proof that God loves us and wants us to be happy"
-unknown

- 8 cups gluten free puffed rice cereal
- 1/3 cup corn syrup
- 1/3 cup butter or margarine
- 1/4 cup brown sugar, packed
- 3 Tbs unsweetened cocoa powder

    Place puffed rice in large bowl, set aside. Grease a 9x9-inch pan. In a large saucepan, place the corn syrup, butter, brown sugar and cocoa. Cook over medium heat, stirring often until mixture comes to a full boil. Boil for 1 minute, remove from heat.
    Pour chocolate mixture over puffed rice cereal and stir with a wooden spoon, making sure it's evenly coated. Press mixture into prepared pan with a spatula. Cool, then cut into squares.

Tip: Store in an airtight container or wrap individually.

-makes 16 bars

Crispy Rice Bars

"Luck is having a rice dumpling fly into your mouth"
-Japanese proverb

- 5 cups gluten free crispy rice cereal
- 1 (10 oz) package large gluten free marshmallows
- 1/2 cup butter or margarine

Place butter in a microwaveable casserole dish. Place in microwave and melt for about 30 seconds. Add marshmallows, cover and cook for 2 to 3 minutes. Remove from microwave and stir until melted and well blended.

Add cereal and stir until well coated. Press warm mixture evenly and firmly into a lightly buttered 8x12-inch pan. Cool, then cut into squares.

-makes 24 bars

Desserts

Easy Cinnamon Buns

"The smell of good buns, like the sound of flowing water is indescribable in it's evocation of innocence and delight"
-M.F.K Fisher (1908-1992)

- 2 cups gluten free pancake mix
- 1/4 cup butter or margarine, softened
- 3 Tbs white sugar
- 2/3 cup milk
- 3 tsp cinnamon
- 1/2 cup raisons

TOPPING:
- 1 cup butter, softened
- 1 1/2 cup corn syrup
- 1 1/2 cup white sugar
- 1/2 tsp salt
- 1 tsp cinnamon
- 1/2 cup chopped nuts, optional

Topping: In a baking dish beat together 1 cup butter, 1 1/2 cup corn syrup, 1 1/2 cup sugar, 1 tsp cinnamon, nuts and salt. Bake at 350°F for 10 minutes. Stir; cool.

Preheat oven to 450°F. Line cookie sheet with parchment paper. Combine 2 cups pancake mix, 3 tsp cinnamon, 1/4 cup butter, 1/2 cup raisons and 3 Tbs sugar. Mix until crumbly, stir in milk. Drop by rounded golf balls onto cookie sheets. Bake 10 minutes. Let cool. Drizzle with topping.

Note: Freeze leftovers same day to maintain freshness.

-6 to 8 buns

Easy Crustless Pumpkin Pie

"No spring nor summer beauty hath such grace as I have seen on one autumnal face"
-John Donne

- 3 eggs, lightly beaten
- 1/3 cup honey
- 1/2 tsp ground ginger
- 1/2 tsp ground nutmeg
- 1/2 tsp ground cinnamon
- 1/2 tsp salt
- 1 1/2 cup cooked pumpkin
- 1 cup evaporated milk, undiluted

Preheat oven to 325°F. Beat eggs slightly. Add honey, ginger, nutmeg, cinnamon, salt and cooked pumpkin. Mix well. Add evaporated milk to pumpkin mixture, stirring to blend.

Pour mixture into a deep, well greased 9-inch pie pan. Bake for 50 to 60 minutes or until set in center. Chill thoroughly before cutting. To serve, cut into pie-shaped wedges, and top with whipped cream.

-6 to 8 servings

Desserts

French Chocolate Cake

"Don't wreck a sublime chocolate experience by feeling guilty"
-Lora Brody

- 1 (8 oz) cup unsalted butter
- 1/2 cup (4 oz) bittersweet baking chocolate, chopped
- 3 eggs
- 1/2 cup unsweetened cocoa powder
- 3/4 cup white sugar

Preheat oven to 300°F. Butter the cake pan, set aside. Coarsely chop the chocolate and melt with butter in a double boiler over simmering water, stirring occasionally. Remove from heat and let cool. In a large bowl beat the eggs at medium speed until thick, about 1 minute. At low speed, beat in the sifted cocoa and then the sugar, to partially blend.

Scrape down sides of bowl with a rubber spatula. Beat mixture at high speed until thick, about 1 minute. Add the melted chocolate and beat at medium speed until blended. Pour into a buttered 8x8-inch cake pan. Bake for around 25 minutes or until done- you can test by using a clean knife- if it comes out clean it's done.

Note: If you wish to turn this cake onto a serving platter, it is a good idea to grease pan and line bottom with greased parchment paper before pouring in batter and baking.

Tip: Serve with whipped cream if desired. This dense, rich cake is also delicious just served plain.

Gingerbread Men

"Had I but a penny in the world, thou shouldst have it for gingerbread"
- William Shakespeare (1564-1616)

- 2 Tbs margarine, softened, not melted
- 2 Tbs cooking molasses
- 2 Tbs white sugar
- 1 tsp ground cinnamon
- 1/2 tsp ground ginger
- 3 Tbs water
- 1 cup gluten free pancake mix

Preheat oven to 275°F. In a large bowl, blend margarine, molasses, sugar, cinnamon and ginger. Stir in 1 cup pancake mix. Slowly add water, kneading until good consistency is reached. Roll out on wax paper 1/4-inch thick. Cut gingerbread men shapes with small cookie cutter. Place on a lightly greased cookie sheet. Bake for 20 to 25 minutes. Remove; let cool slightly then transfer to wire rack to completely cool. Decorate as desired.

Tip: To save time, you could simply roll the dough into small balls and flatten with a fork or flat bottomed bowl, then bake.

Note: Store frozen to maintain freshness.

-makes about 12 small gingerbread men

Desserts

Graham Cracker Cookies

"Animal crackers and cocoa to drink, that is the finest of suppers I think"
		-Christopher Morley

- 2 Tbs margarine
- 2 Tbs liquid honey
- 2 Tbs white sugar
- 1/2 tsp gluten free vanilla extract
- 1 cup gluten free pancake mix
- 3 Tbs water
- ground cinnamon to taste

Preheat oven to 275°F. Blend together the margarine, sugar, honey and vanilla in a large bowl. Add pancake mix, cut in with fork. Add water a little at a time, to form a cookie dough consistency. Roll the dough into walnut sized balls.
Place on a lightly greased cookie sheet. Use a flat bottomed bowl to flatten each. Sprinkle with cinnamon if desired. Bake for 20 to 25 minutes or until golden brown.

Note: Store in freezer to maintain freshness. These are not exactly like real graham crackers, but close enough.

Tip: You could use these to make Smores, or finely crush into crumbs for use in recipes requiring graham cracker crumbs.

-makes about 12 round graham cracker cookies

Gourmet Dark Chocolate Cookies

"The 12- step chocoholics program: never be more than 12 steps away from chocolate"
-Terry Moore

- 3/4 cup unsweetened cocoa powder
- 2 1/2 cups gluten free icing sugar
- 1/2 tsp salt
- 2 cups chopped walnuts, or nuts of choice
- 1 Tbs gluten free vanilla extract
- 4 egg whites

Preheat the oven to 350°F. Put everything except the egg whites and vanilla into a large bowl and mix with a wooden spoon for 1 minute. In a separate bowl, combine the vanilla and egg whites. Add this to the dry mixture. With a mixer on medium speed, blend everything for 2 minutes.

Scoop the dough-it will be runny-by heaping teaspoons onto a parchment paper lined cookie sheet, or these cookies stick. Space cookies a few inches apart, as they spread a lot while baking. Lower the oven temperature to 320°F and bake for 8 minutes or until small cracks appear on the surface. Cool slightly then very carefully transfer them to a wire rack to finish cooling. These cookies will have a nice, shiny glaze.

Note: These can be stored in a regular cookie jar without fear of drying out.

Desserts

Individual Frozen Cheesecakes

"Individuality is freedom lived"
         -John Dos Passos

- 3/4 cup finely ground nuts
- 1 Tbs butter, melted
- 1 envelope gluten free unflavored gelatin
- 1/4 cup cold water
- 1 1/2 cups (12 oz) cream cheese
- 1/3 cup white sugar
- 3/4 cup milk
- 1/4 tsp gluten free vanilla extract

Combine finely ground nuts and butter in a bowl. Press into bottom of 12 paper-lined muffin cups. Cover; freeze for 10 minutes. Meanwhile, in a small saucepan, sprinkle gelatin over cold water and let stand for 1 minute. Cook on low heat, stirring until gelatin is dissolved and set aside. In a mixing bowl, beat cream cheese and sugar. Gradually beat in milk and vanilla. Stir in gelatin mixture. Spoon into muffin cups; freeze until firm.

Remove desserts 10 minutes before serving. Peel liners off desserts and invert onto individual plates (crust sides up). Drizzle with melted chocolate, or gluten free fruit pie filling, or a raspberry puree, or whatever you like. Garnish with berries if desired.

-12 servings

Mini Cream Cheese Coconut Bites

"If you cannot do great things, do small things in a great way"
-Napoleon Hill

- 1 (8 oz) package cream cheese, softened
- 1/2 cup smooth gluten free peanut butter
- 1/4 cup white sugar
- 1/4 tsp ground cinnamon
- 1/4 tsp gluten free vanilla extract
- 1 cup unsweetened shredded coconut
- 1/4 cup finely ground nuts
- unsweetened shredded coconut for coating

In a medium bowl, with electric mixer on medium speed, combine the softened cream cheese, peanut butter, sugar, cinnamon, vanilla, 1 cup shredded coconut and finely ground nuts, scraping down sides of bowl as needed. Chill 60 minutes or until firm.

Roll into 3/4-inch balls, then roll in shredded coconut. Chill for an additional 15 minutes minimum before serving.

Note: these are nice at Christmas time as they look like little snowballs.

-30 bite size cheesecake treats

Desserts

5 Minute Chocolate Cake

"Lost time is never found again"
-Benjamin Franklin

- 3 Tbs finely ground nuts
- 3 Tbs rice flour
- 1 Tbs unsweetened baking cocoa
- 1/4 Tbs gluten free baking powder
- 2 Tbs liquid honey
- 2 Tbs butter or margarine, melted
- 1 Tbs water
- 1 egg

In a 2-cup pyrex baking dish blend together well the powdered nuts, rice flour, cocoa, baking powder and honey. Add water, egg and melted margarine. Blend thoroughly with fork. Cover with plastic wrap, cut small slit to vent. Microwave on high for 1 minute then check to see if done. If more time is required continue cooking checking every 30 seconds. It is done when a knife comes out clean. Cooking time will vary with microwaves, anywhere from 1 to 3 minutes bake time required. Over cooking will dry out the cake. Turn onto plate to cool.

Note: This is a spongy, not very sweet cake that tastes best if served frosted or with whipped cream. You could also drizzle with a chocolate ganache (cream and chocolate melted together to form a sauce).

-2 to 4 servings

Mocha Brownies

"Enjoy the little things, for one day you may look back and realize they were the big things"
-Robert Brault

- 5 squares gluten free semi-sweet baking chocolate
- 1/2 cup butter or margarine
- 1 tsp gluten free vanilla extract
- 1 tsp strongly brewed black coffee
- 1 cup finely ground nuts
- 3 oz (1/3 cup) liquid honey
- 4 eggs, separated

Preheat oven to 350°F. Grease an 8-inch square pan and line the bottom with parchment paper, also greased. Melt the chocolate and butter together in microwave for about one minute, then a little longer until melted and smooth. Stir in the coffee and vanilla. Leave to cool slightly, then add the nuts and honey, mixing well until combined. Separate the eggs. Beat the egg yolks lightly then stir them into the prepared chocolate.

Whip the egg whites until they form stiff peaks. Fold into the chocolate mixture, blending until completely mixed in. Spoon mixture into the prepared pan and bake for 20 to 25 minutes until firm on top but still slightly gooey in center. Let cool in pan, then turn out, removing parchment and cut into pieces.

-16 servings

Desserts

Mom's Sweet Marie Bars

"My mother had a great deal of trouble with me but I think she enjoyed it"
-Mark Twain

- 1 cup light brown sugar
- 1 cup corn syrup
- 1 cup gluten free peanut butter
- 2 tsp gluten free vanilla extract
- 2 Tbs butter or margarine, softened not melted
- 5 cups gluten free crispy rice cereal

ICING:
- 1/2 package gluten free chocolate chips or gluten free butterscotch morsels

Combine brown sugar, corn syrup and peanut butter in a large pan over medium heat, stirring until well blended. Do not boil. Remove from heat and add vanilla and butter. Stir in crispy rice cereal. Press into a well-buttered 9x9-inch pan. Refrigerate. Cut into 1-inch squares. Melt chocolate chips in double boiler, stir, spread over bars.

Note: you can use any icing you prefer in place of melted chips. You can freeze these bars, but if you do and want to frost them, do so after they are removed from the freezer. I have also made these with crushed gluten free corn flake cereal in place of the crispy rice cereal, with good results.

Nanaimo Bars

"I can resist anything except temptation"
Oscar Wilde

LAYER 1:
- 1/2 cup butter or margarine
- 1/4 cup white sugar
- 5 Tbs unsweetened cocoa
- 1 egg, beaten
- 1 3/4 cups gluten free graham cracker crumbs
- 3/4 cup fine or medium shredded coconut
- 1/2 cup finely chopped walnuts

LAYER 2:
- 1/2 cup butter or margarine
- 3 Tbs milk
- 2 Tbs vanilla custard powder
- 2 cups gluten free icing sugar

LAYER 3:
- 2/3 cup gluten free semi-sweet chocolate chips
- 2 Tbs butter or margarine

Layer 1: Melt first 3 ingredients over medium heat. Add beaten egg and stir to cook and thicken. Remove from heat. Stir in crumbs, coconut and nuts. Press into non-greased 9x9-inch pan.

Layer 2: Blend butter, icing sugar, milk and custard powder in a bowl until smooth. Spread over 1st layer.

Layer 3: Melt chocolate and butter over low heat, careful not to over cook. Spread over second layer. Chill until firm. Use a sharp knife to cut into squares.

Desserts

Ooey-Gooey Raspberry Chocolate Cakes

"Research tells us fourteen out of any ten individuals likes chocolate"
                    -Sandra Boynton

- 8 oz (250g) semi-sweet baking chocolate, chopped
- 1/2 cup butter or margarine
- 2/3 cup white sugar
- 3 eggs, at room temperature
- 2 tsp gluten free vanilla extract
- 1/4 cup white rice flour
- 1/4 cup unsweetened cocoa powder
- 1/4 tsp ground cinnamon
- 18 fresh or frozen raspberries

Preheat oven to 375°F. Grease 6 cup large muffin tin. Melt chocolate in a heat safe bowl, placed over a pot of barely simmering water, stirring often. Remove. In another bowl, beat butter and sugar until smooth. Add eggs one at a time, beating well after each addition. Stir in vanilla and cooled chocolate. Blend in rice flour, cocoa and cinnamon.

Spoon mixture into greased muffin cups. Press 3 raspberries into center of each cake and spread filling to make level. Bake for 12 to 15 minutes, just until tops of cakes lose their shine. Let cool for 2 minutes, then very carefully remove and serve on individual plates. These cakes have wonderful gooey centers.

Tip: Batter can be made in advance and chilled, just add an extra 3 minutes to bake time.

- 6 individual "molten lava" cakes

Peanut Butter Chocolate Chip Cookies

"Broken cookies don't have calories"
-unknown

- 1/2 cup margarine
- 3/4 cup gluten free peanut butter
- 1 cup white rice flour
- 1/4 cup tapioca flour
- 2 Tbs xanthum gum
- 1/2 cup white sugar
- 1/2 cup brown sugar, packed
- one large egg
- 1/2 tsp baking soda
- 1/2 tsp gluten free baking powder
- 1/4 cup water
- 1 (300g) bag gluten free chocolate chips

In a bowl beat margarine and peanut butter with an electric mixer until blended well. Add rice flour, tapioca flour, sugars, egg, baking soda, baking powder, and xanthum gum. Beat until combined well. Add 1/4 cup of water, a little at a time, kneading with hands, until a good cookie dough consistency is reached. You may not need to use all the water.

Preheat oven to 375°F. Shape into 1-inch balls, and flatten slightly. Place on non-stick cookie sheets and bake for around 12 to 15 minutes or until lightly browned . Let cool for a couple minutes, before transferring to wire rack to finish cooling. Store frozen.

- 3 1/2 dozen cookies

Desserts

Peanut Butter Cinnamon Cookies

"A balanced diet is a cookie in each hand"
-Barbara Johnson

- 2 cups gluten free peanut butter
- 2 cups white sugar
- 2 eggs
- 1 tsp cinnamon
- 1/2 tsp gluten free vanilla extract, optional

Preheat oven to 350°F. Combine all ingredients well. Drop by the teaspoonful onto a non-greased cookie sheet. Bake for about 8 minutes. Let cool.

Note: For "peanut butter and jelly" cookies omit the cinnamon and vanilla . Make small holes on top of each and fill with jam (not jelly, it melts) before baking.

Tip: You could dip these cookies in melted chocolate and crushed nuts if desired.

-about 24 cookies

Peanut Butter Crispy Rice Bars

"A loving heart is the truest wisdom"
-Charles Dickens

- 2/3 cup sweetened condensed milk (NOT evaporated milk)
- 1/4 cup gluten free peanut butter
- 1/4 cup light corn syrup
- 1/2 cup brown sugar, packed
- 4 cups gluten free crispy rice cereal

ICING:
- 1/2 cup gluten free chocolate chips
- 2 Tbs peanut butter

Over medium-low heat cook condensed milk, peanut butter, corn syrup and brown sugar in a sauce pan until well mixed and thickened, stirring constantly. Remove from heat. Add cereal stirring to coat.

Grease a 9x9-inch pan. Firmly press rice mixture into pan. Cool. Melt chocolate chips and peanut butter over low heat and spread over bars. Cut into squares.

-25 servings

Desserts

Pots De Creme

"It's kind of fun to do the impossible"
-Walt Disney

- 4 oz semi-sweet baking chocolate
- 2 Tbs white sugar
- 3/4 cup light cream
- 2 egg yolks, slightly beaten
- 1/2 tsp gluten free vanilla extract

In a medium sauce pan, heat chocolate, sugar, and cream over medium heat, stirring constantly until the chocolate is melted and the mixture is smooth.

Remove from heat; gradually beat into egg yolks. Blend in vanilla. Pour into small serving dishes. Chill well before serving.

-4 to 6 servings

Rocky Road Pudding

"Our way is not soft grass, it is a rocky mountain path, but it goes forwards; upwards, toward the sun"
-unknown

- 1/2 cup white sugar
- 5 Tbs unsweetened cocoa
- 3 Tbs corn starch or potato starch
- 1/8 tsp salt
- 2 1/2 cups milk
- 2 egg yolks, lightly beaten
- 2 tsp gluten free vanilla extract
- 1 cup gluten free miniature marshmallows
- 1/4 cup chopped nuts, toasted

In a large sauce pan, combine the sugar, cocoa, cornstarch and salt. Stir in milk until smooth. Cook over high heat, stirring constantly until thickened and bubbly. Reduce heat; cook and stir 2 minutes longer. Remove from heat. Stir a small amount of hot filling into egg yolks; return all to the pan, stirring constantly. Bring to a gentle boil; cook and stir for 2 minutes.

Remove from heat. Gently stir in vanilla. Cool for 15 minutes, stirring occasionally. Transfer to individual dessert dishes. Cover and refrigerate for 1 hour. Top with nuts and marshmallows before serving.

-5 servings

Desserts

Shortbread Cookies

"I am not a glutton- I am an explorer of food"
Erma Bombeck

- 1/2 cup cornstarch
- 1/2 cup gluten free icing sugar
- 1 cup white rice flour
- 3/4 cup margarine
- 2 tsp xanthum gum or 4 tsp unflavored gelatin

Sift cornstarch, sugar, xanthum gum and rice flour together in bowl. Add margarine and mix with hands until soft dough forms. Refrigerate for one hour.

Preheat oven to 300°F. Shape chilled dough into 1-inch balls, then flatten slightly. Place on a lightly greased cookie sheet spaced about 1-inch apart.

Bake for 20 to 25 minutes or until edges are lightly golden. Let cool. Store frozen. Frost if desired.

-2 dozen cookies

Whole Orange Cake

"A man ought to carry himself in the world as an orange tree would if it could walk up and down in the garden, swinging perfume from every little censer it holds up to the air"
-Henry Ward Beecher (1813-1887)

- 2 whole oranges, peels on, preferably seedless
- 2 1/2 cups (250 g) almonds, finely ground to powder
- 1 cup superfine sugar
- 1 tsp gluten free baking powder
- 6 eggs

Boil two whole oranges, peels on, for 1 1/2 to 2 hours, then puree in blender. Meanwhile, in a bowl combine the almond powder, sugar and baking powder. Set aside. Add the eggs to the oranges, and blend. Pour orange puree into the dry mix, stirring to blend.

Grease parchment paper and line an 8x8-inch cake pan. Pour in batter. Bake at 350°F for about 60 minutes. Turn out onto a plate when cooled. Frost if desired.

Note: This wonderfully moist cake tastes even better after a few days. It stays fresh in refrigerator for weeks. Lemons could be substituted to make a "lemon cake."

Desserts

Yummy Peanut Butter Balls

"Peanut butter is the pate' of childhood"
-Florence Fabricant

- 1 Tbs butter or margarine
- 1/3 cup gluten free smooth peanut butter
- 1 cup gluten free icing sugar
- 4 squares semi-sweet baking chocolate

Line a cookie sheet with wax paper, set aside. Mix together the butter, peanut butter and icing sugar. Form into 1-inch balls. Melt the chocolate, being careful not to overcook.
Remove from heat. Roll peanut butter balls in the heated chocolate, evenly coating. Set on prepared cookie sheet to firm, then store in airtight container.

Tip: You could get creative with these, and roll them in shredded coconut, nuts, gluten free sprinkles, or whatever you like.

Miscellaneous

Miscellaneous

Baked English Omelette

"To eat well in England you should have breakfast three times a day"
-W. Somerset Maugham

- 6 eggs, beaten
- 2/3 cup milk
- 1/4 tsp salt
- 1/8 tsp pepper
- 1 1/2 cups cheddar cheese, shredded
- 1 green onion, thinly sliced
- 3 slices bacon, cooked and crumbled
- 1 Tbs butter or margarine
- 1 Tbs fresh parmesan

Preheat oven to 400°F. In large bowl, beat milk into eggs. Stir in seasonings, cheddar, green onion and bacon. Melt butter and pour into egg mixture.

Pour into casserole dish and sprinkle with parmesan. Bake for 20 minutes or until set and lightly golden. Serve immediately.

-2 to 3 servings

Chocolate Icing

"If you're going to lick the icing off somebody else's cake you won't be nourished and it won't do you any good"
-Emily Carr

- 2/3 cup butter, unsalted
- 1 3/4 cups gluten free icing sugar
- 1/4 cup unsweetened cocoa, sifted
- 1 to 2 Tbs hot water

Melt the butter in a pan. Add the icing sugar and cocoa powder and blend well. Add 1 to 2 Tbs hot water and beat until glossy.

Refrigerate for 15 minutes or until the icing has a spreadable consistency. Use to frost a cooled cake or cup cakes.

Miscellaneous

Coconut Pecan Frosting

"A cheerful look makes a dish a feast"
　　　　　　　　　　-George Herbert

- 1 cup white sugar
- 1 cup evaporated milk
- 1/2 cup butter
- 3 eggs, beaten
- 1 1/3 cup flaked coconut
- 1 cup chopped pecans or walnuts
- 1 tsp gluten free vanilla extract

In a medium sauce pan, combine 1 cup sugar, evaporated milk, 1/2 cup butter and 3 beaten eggs. Cook over medium heat until mixture starts to bubble, stirring constantly.

Remove from heat. Stir in coconut, nuts and vanilla. Cool until room temperature. Spread on a cooled cake.

Cream Cheese Frosting

"Eating words has never given me indigestion"
-Winston Churchill (1874-1965)

- 1 (8 oz) package of cream cheese, room temperature
- 2 cups gluten free icing sugar
- 2 tsp gluten free vanilla extract
- 1 Tbs butter, softened, not melted

Cream the cream cheese until softened. Add softened butter, icing sugar and vanilla extract.

Beat until well blended and smooth. Spread on cooled cake or cup cakes.

Miscellaneous

Easy Breakfast For One

"An egg is always an adventure; the next one may be different"
-Oscar Wilde

- 1 slice gluten free bread, toasted
- 1 tsp butter or margarine
- 3 fresh mushrooms, thinly sliced
- 3 tomato slices
- 2 Tbs grated parmesan cheese
- 1 slice crisply cooked bacon, crumbled

Preheat oven to 350°F. Place toast on baking sheet. Spread with butter if desired.
Cover with mushrooms and tomato slices. Sprinkle cheese and crumbled bacon on top. Bake until cheese melts.

-1 serving

French Toast

"All happiness depends on a leisurely breakfast"
-John Gunther

- 3 eggs
- 1/2 tsp salt
- 2 Tbs white sugar
- 1 cup milk
- 6 slices gluten free bread
- ground cinnamon to taste
- gluten free maple syrup

In a large bowl, beat eggs; add salt, sugar and milk. Mix well. Dip gluten free bread in mixture until completely covered.

Cook in a greased, hot frying pan or griddle. Brown on one side, turn and brown the other side. Serve hot sprinkled with cinnamon and drizzled with syrup.

-3 to 6 servings

Miscellaneous

Mozzarella And Bacon Frittata

"He that looketh on a plate of ham and eggs to lust after it hath already committed breakfast with it in his heart"
-C.S. Lewis (1898-1963)

- 8 eggs
- 2 tablespoons water
- 1/2 cup tomato, chopped and seeded
- 1 cup mozzarella cheese. divided
- 2 tablespoons real bacon bits
- 1/2 cup fresh basil, chopped

Preheat oven to 350°F. Beat eggs and water with wire whisk in a medium bowl. Stir in tomato, 1/2 cup of cheese, bacon bits and basil. Pour into 9 - inch pie plate and sprinkle with remaining half cup of cheese. Bake for 30 minutes or until puffed and golden brown.

Note: For a Spinach and Mushroom version, substitute the basil with spinach, the bacon with mushrooms, and the mozzarella with cheddar cheese.

-4 servings

Toasted Pumpkin Seeds

"High-tech tomatoes. Super squash. Are we supposed to eat this stuff? Or is it going to eat us?"
- Annita Manning

- 1 medium sized pumpkin
- Olive Oil
- Salt

Preheat oven to 400°F. Cut open pumpkin, and, using a strong metal spoon, scrape out the insides. Separate the seeds from the stringy core and rinse the seeds.

In a small saucepan, add the seeds to water, about 2 cups of water to every 1/2 cup of seeds. Add a tablespoon of salt for every cup of water. Bring to a boil then let simmer for about 10 minutes. Remove from heat and drain.

Use olive oil to grease a cookie sheet. Spread seeds on the sheet in one layer. Bake on the top rack for 20 minutes or until seeds begin to brown. Remove, and let fully cool before eating.

Index

Appetizers
Baked Potato Skins - 8
Cheddar Cheese Ball - 9
Cheese Nacho's - 10
Chicken Fingers - 11
Deli Meat Roll-ups - 12
Deviled Eggs - 13
Holiday Cheese Truffles - 14
Honey Mustard Chicken
       Wings - 15
Parmesan Hummus Dip - 16
Smoked Salmon Spread - 17
Spinach Artichoke Dip - 18

Beverages
Christmas Party Punch - 20
Cranberry Ginger Tea - 21
Fountain of Youth Smoothie - 22
Iced Cappuccino - 23
Mimosa - 24
Mochaccino - 25
Orange Smoothie - 26
Peanut Butter Banana
    Smoothie - 27
Peppermint Hot Chocolate - 28
Pina Colada - 29
Raspberry Iced Tea - 30

Soups
Clam Chowder - 32
Hearty Hamburger Soup - 33
Mom's Chicken Soup - 34
Mushroom Soup - 35
Potato Leak Soup - 36
Vegetarian Bean Soup - 37
Yummy Tomato Basil Soup - 38

Salads
Black Bean Salad - 40
Chef Salad - 41
Cranberry Pecan Salad - 42
Crunchy Coleslaw - 43
Easy Greek Salad - 44
Fruit & Cheese Summer Salad - 45
Marinated Veggie Salad - 46
Popeyes' Spinach Salad - 47
Potato Salad - 48

Side Dishes
Asparagus With Lemon Butter - 50
Cheesy Rice Casserole - 51
Coconut Almond Broccoli - 52
Cream Corn - 53
Crunchy Pecan Wild Rice - 54
Delicious Rice Stuffing - 55
Oven Roasted New Potatoes - 56
Stuffed Baked Potatoes - 57
Sunshine Carrots - 58
Sweet Potatoes - 59
The Best Mashed Potatoes - 60
Zucchini For Two - 61
Zucchini Parmesan - 62

Gluten Free & Fabulous

Entrees
Adams' Ribs - 64
Apple Cinnamon Chicken - 65
Baked Spicy Sweet Ham - 66
Barbecue Tenderloin Steaks - 67
Brown Sugar Chicken - 68
Cheese Stuffed Chicken - 69
Crock Pot Apple Pork Roast - 70
Easy Chili - 71
Grilled Lemon Oregano Fish - 72
Herbed Salmon Steaks - 73
Honey Garlic Chicken - 74
Lemon Parsley Halibut - 75
Manhattan Meatballs - 76
Maple Syrup Chicken - 77
Orange Zest Salmon - 78
Oven-Crisped Pork Chops - 79
Parmesan Chicken - 80
Pineapple chicken - 81
Simple Sweet & Sour Chops - 82
Spiced Chicken - 83
Sweet & Spicy Chicken - 84
Tarragon Chicken - 85
Yummy Lasagna Casserole - 86

Baked Goods
Brazilian Cheese Buns - 88
Corn Muffins - 89
Cheesy Pizza Crust - 90
Potato Flat Bread - 91
Simply Nutty Banana Bread - 92

Desserts
Almond Pecan Cake - 94
Apple Crumble - 95
Babe Ruth Bars - 96
Baked Cinnamon Apples - 97
Basic Cheesecake - 98
Berry Lemon Mousse Parfait - 99
Caramel Bananas - 100
Chocolate Almond Cupcakes - 101
Chocolate Cake Cookies - 102
Chocolate Cake Pudding - 103
Chocolate Chip Cookies - 104
Chocolate Dipped Ice Cream - 105
Chocolate Dipped Pecan
   Bites - 106
Chocolate Marshmallow
   Truffles - 107
Chocolate Mousse Pie - 108
Chocolate Peanut Cups - 109
Chocolate Puffed Rice
   Squares - 110
Crispy Rice Bars - 111
Easy Cinnamon Buns - 112
Easy Crustless Pumpkin Pie - 113
French Chocolate Cake - 114
Ginger Bread Men - 115
Graham Cracker Cookies - 116
Gourmet Chocolate Cookies - 117
Individual Frozen Cheesecakes - 118
Mini Cream Cheese Coconut
   Bites - 119
5 Minute Chocolate Cake - 120
Mocha Brownies - 121
Moms' Sweet Marie Bars - 122
Nanaimo Bars - 123
Ooey-Gooey Raspberry Chocolate
   Cakes - 124

Peanut Butter Chocolate Chip
Cookies - 125
Peanut Butter Cinnamon
    Cookies - 126
Peanut Butter Crispy
    Rice Bars - 127
Pots De Creme - 128
Rocky Road Pudding - 129
Shortbread Cookies - 130
Whole Orange Cake - 131
Yummy Peanut Butter Balls - 132

Miscellaneous
Baked English Omelette - 134
Chocolate Icing - 135
Coconut Pecan Frosting - 136
Cream Cheese Frosting - 137
Easy Breakfast For One - 138
French Toast - 139
Mozzarella & Bacon Frittata - 140
Toasted Pumpkin Seeds - 141

"Challenges are what make life interesting; overcoming them is what makes life meaningful"
    -Joshua J. Marine

Printed in the United States
65965LVS00009B/49